Advances in Intestinal Transplantation, Part I

Editor

ALAN L. BUCHMAN

GASTROENTEROLOGY CLINICS OF NORTH AMERICA

www.gastro.theclinics.com

Consulting Editor
ALAN L. BUCHMAN

June 2024 • Volume 53 • Number 2

ELSEVIER

1600 John F. Kennedy Boulevard • Suite 1800 • Philadelphia, Pennsylvania, 19103-2899

http://www.theclinics.com

GASTROENTEROLOGY CLINICS OF NORTH AMERICA Volume 53, Number 2
June 2024 ISSN 0889-8553, ISBN-13: 978-0-443-12981-0

Editor: Kerry Holland
Developmental Editor: Malvika Shah

Gastroenterology Clinics of North America (ISSN 0889-8553) is published quarterly by Elsevier Inc., 360 Park Avenue South, New York, NY 10010-1710. Months of issue are March, June, September, and December. Business and Editorial Offices: 1600 John F. Kennedy Blvd., Suite 1800, Philadelphia, PA 19103-2899. Customer Service Office: 6277 Sea Harbor Drive, Orlando, FL 32887-4800. Periodicals postage paid at New York, NY and additional mailing offices. Subscription prices are $387.00 per year (US individuals), $100.00 per year (US students), $407.00 per year (Canadian individuals), $100.00 per year (Canadian students), $496.00 per year (international individuals), $220.00 per year (international students). For institutional access pricing please contact Customer Service via the contact information below. Foreign air speed delivery is included in all *Clinics* subscription prices. All prices are subject to change without notice. **POSTMASTER**: Send address changes to *Gastroenterology Clinics of North America*, Elsevier Health Sciences Division, Subscription Customer Service, 3251 Riverport Lane, Maryland Heights, MO 63043. **Telephone: 1-800-654-2452 (U.S. and Canada); 314-447-8871 (outside U.S. and Canada). Fax: 314-447-8029. E-mail: journalscustomerservice-usa@elsevier.com (for print support); journalsonlinesupport-usa@elsevier.com (for online support).**

Reprints. For copies of 100 or more, of articles in this publication, please contact the Commercial Reprints Department, Elsevier Inc., 360 Part Avenue South, New York, New York 10010-1710. Tel. 212-633-3874, Fax: 212-633-3820, E-mail: reprints@elsevier.com.

Gastroenterology Clinics of North America is also published in Italian by Il Pensiero Scientifico Editore, Rome, Italy; and in Portuguese by Interlivros Edicoes Ltda., Rua Commandante Coelho 1085, 21250 Cordovil, Rio de Janeiro, Brazil.

Gastroenterology Clinics of North America is covered in *MEDLINE/PubMed (Index Medicus), Excerpta Medica, Current Contents/Clinical Medicine, Science Citation Index, ISI/BIOMED*, and *BIOSIS*.

Printed in the United States of America.

Contributors

CONSULTING EDITOR

ALAN L. BUCHMAN, MD, MSPH, FACP, FACN, FACG, AGAF
Professor of Clinical Surgery, Medical Director, Intestinal Rehabilitation and Transplant Center, The University of Illinois at Chicago, UI Health/Chicago, Illinois, USA

EDITOR

ALAN L. BUCHMAN, MD, MSPH, FACP, FACN, FACG, AGAF
Professor of Clinical Surgery, Medical Director, Intestinal Rehabilitation and Transplant Center, The University of Illinois at Chicago, UI Health/Chicago, Illinois, USA

AUTHORS

ENRICO BENEDETTI, MD
Professor, Division of Transplantation, Department of Surgery, University of Illinois at Chicago, Chicago, Illinois, USA

DANA LIZA BOCTOR, MD, FRCPC, MSc
Section of Gastroenterology, Hepatology and Nutrition, Alberta Children's Hospital, University of Calgary, Calgary, Alberta, Canada

GEOFFREY JAMES BOND, MD
Assistant Professor in Transplant Surgery, Thomas E. Starzl Transplantation Institute, Children's Hospital of Pittsburgh of UPMC, University of Pittsburgh, Pittsburgh, Pennsylvania, USA

LAURENS J. CEULEMANS, MD, PhD
Professor, Department of Thoracic Surgery, Leuven Intestinal Failure and Transplantation (LIFT) Center, Department of Chronic Diseases and Metabolism, Laboratory of Respiratory Diseases and Thoracic Surgery (BREATHE), KU Leuven, University Hospitals Leuven, Leuven, Belgium

NATHALIE P. DEFERM, MD
Abdominal Surgeon, Department of General and Abdominal Surgery, Sint-Franciscus Hospital, Heusden-Zolder, Belgium

PIERPAOLO DI COCCO, MD, PhD
Assistant Professor, Division of Transplantation, Department of Surgery, University of Illinois at Chicago, Chicago, Illinois, USA

RAFAEL MIYASHIRO NUNES DOS SANTOS, MD
Assistant Professor of Surgery, Transplant, UMMG Department of Surgery, Miller School of Medicine, Medical Campus, University of Miami, Miami, Florida, USA

ANTOINE DUBOIS, MD
PhD Candidate, Department of Microbiology, Immunology and Transplantation, KU Leuven, Leuven Intestinal Failure and Transplantation (LIFT) Center, Department of Abdominal Transplant Surgery, University Hospitals Leuven, Leuven, Belgium

TANIS R. FENTON, RD, PhD
Adjunct Professor, Cumming School of Medicine, University of Calgary Nutrition Services, Alberta Health Services, Department of Community Health Sciences, Institute of Public Health, Alberta Children's Hospital Research Institute, Calgary, Alberta, Canada

JENNIFER GARCIA, MD
Associate Professor, UMMG Department of Pediatrics, Miller School of Medicine, Medical Campus, University of Miami, Miami, Florida, USA

OLIVIER GOULET, MD, PhD
Chairman and Professor, Department of Pediatric Gastroenterology, Hepatology and Nutrition, University of Paris Medical School, National Reference Center for Rare Digestive Diseases, Pediatric Intestinal Failure Rehabilitation Center, Hô pital Necker-Enfants Malades, Paris, France

INA HENNION, MSc
Tissue Engineering Lab, Department of Development and Regeneration, KU Leuven, KULAK Campus Kortrijk, Kortrijk, Belgium

JUDY HOPKINS, OTD, OT/L, SWC
Occupational Therapist, Division of Occupational Therapy, Children's Hospital Los Angeles, Los Angeles, California, USA

KISHORE R. IYER, MBBS, FRCS (ENG), FACS
Professor of Surgery, Pediatrics and Global Health, Director, Intestinal Rehabilitation and Transplant Program, Icahn School of Medicine at Mount Sinai, Mount Sinai Hospital, New York, New York, USA

JESS JOHNSON, BS
MD Candidate, University of Illinois at Chicago College of Medicine, Chicago, Illinois, USA

TOMOAKI KATO, MD, MBA, FACS
Chief, Division of Abdominal Organ Transplant and Hepatobiliary Surgery, Center for Liver Disease and Transplantation, Columbia University Irving Medical Center, New York, New York, USA

JOSEPH M. LADOWSKI, MD, PhD
Research Fellow, Department of Surgery, Duke University Medical Center, Durham, North Carolina, USA

CECILE LAMBE, MD
Department of Pediatric Gastroenterology, Hepatology and Nutrition, National Reference Center for Rare Digestive Diseases, Pediatric Intestinal Failure Rehabilitation Center, Hôpital Necker-Enfants Malades, University of Paris Medical School, Paris, France

AMY LIAN, BS
MD Candidate, University of Illinois at Chicago College of Medicine, Chicago, Illinois, USA

ALESSANDRO MARTININO, MD
Research Scholar, Division of Transplantation, Department of Surgery, University of Illinois at Chicago, Chicago, Illinois, USA

REI MATSUMOTO, MD, PhD
Intestinal Transplant Research Fellow, Center for Liver Disease and Transplantation, Columbia University Irving Medical Center, New York, New York, USA

RUSSELL MERRITT, MD, PhD
Clinical Professor, Department of Pediatrics, Keck School of Medicine, Pediatric Gastroenterologist, Division of Gastroenterology, Hepatology and Nutrition, Children's Hospital Los Angeles, University of Southern California, Los Angeles, California, USA

EWOUT MUYLLE, BSc
Department of Chronic Diseases and Metabolism, Laboratory of Respiratory Diseases and Thoracic Surgery (BREATHE), KU Leuven, Leuven Intestinal Failure and Transplantation (LIFT) Center, Department of Abdominal Transplant Surgery, University Hospitals Leuven, Leuven, Belgium

BRENT J. PFEIFFER, MD
Assistant Professor of Pediatrics, Critical Care Medicine, UMMG Department of Pediatrics, Miller School of Medicine, Medical Campus, University of Miami, Miami, Florida, USA

JACQUES PIRENNE, MD, PhD
Professor, Faculty of Medicine, Department of Microbiology, Immunology and Transplantation, KU Leuven, Leuven Intestinal Failure and Transplantation (LIFT) Center, Department of Abdominal Transplant Surgery, University Hospitals Leuven, Leuven, Belgium

GENNARO SELVAGGI, MD
Associate Professor of Surgery, Transplant, DeWitt Daughtry Family Department of Surgery, University of Miami, Miami, Florida, USA

MARIO SPAGGIARI, MD
Associate Professor, Division of Transplantation, Department of Surgery, University of Illinois at Chicago, Chicago, Illinois, USA

DEBRA L. SUDAN, MD
Division Chief of Abdominal Transplant, Professor, Department of Surgery, Duke Transplant Center, Duke University School of Medicine, Durham, North Carolina, USA

AKIN TEKIN, MD
Professor of Surgery, Transplant, UMMG Department of Surgery, Miller School of Medicine, Medical Campus, University of Miami, Miami, Florida, USA

LIEVEN THORREZ, PhD
Tissue Engineering Lab, Department of Development and Regeneration, KU Leuven, KULAK Campus Kortrijk, Kortrijk, Belgium

IVO TZVETANOV, MD
Professor, Division of Transplantation, Department of Surgery, University of Illinois at Chicago, Chicago, Illinois, USA

NELE VAN DE WINKEL, MD
Leuven Intestinal Failure and Transplantation (LIFT) Center, Department of Abdominal Surgery, University Hospitals Leuven, Department of Development and Regeneration, Unit of Urogenital, Abdominal and Plastic Surgery, KU Leuven, Leuven, Belgium

VIGHNESH VETRIVEL VENKATASAMY, MD
Assistant Professor of Surgery, Transplant, DeWitt Daughtry Family Department of Surgery, University of Miami, Miami, Florida, USA

RODRIGO M. VIANNA, MD
Professor of Surgery, Transplant, DeWitt Daughtry Family Department of Surgery, University of Miami, Miami, Florida, USA

Contents

> Intestinal allotransplantation was first described in the 1960s and success-fully performed in the 1980s. Since that time, less progress has been made in the preservation of the allograft before transplantation and static cold storage remains the current standard. Normothermic machine perfusion represents an opportunity to simultaneously preserve, assess, and recon-dition the organ for transplantation and improve the procurement radius for allografts. The substantial progress made in the field during the last 60 years, coupled with the success of the preclinical animal model of ma-chine perfusion-preserved intestinal transplantation, suggest we are ap-proaching the point of clinical application.

> Outcomes for patients with chronic intestinal failure have improved with organization of experts into multidisciplinary teams delivering care in intes-tinal rehabilitation programs. There have been improvements in under-standing of intestinal failure complications as well as development of newer therapies that have amplified the improvements in survival. In spite of this encouraging trend, patients who fail PN are often referred too late for intestinal transplantation. The author proposes a more rational frame-work that might allow earlier identification of intestinal failure patients at risk for PN-failure, who could appropriately be considered earlier for intes-tinal transplantation with improvements in overall outcomes.

> Consensus remains elusive in the definition and indications of multivisceral transplantation (MVT) within the transplant community. MVT encompasses transplantation of all organs reliant on the celiac artery axis and the supe-rior mesenteric artery in different combinations. Some institutions classify MVT as involving the grafting of the stomach or ascending colon in addi-tion to the jejunoileal complex. MVT indications span a wide spectrum of conditions, including tumors, intestinal dysmotility disorders, and trauma. This systematic review aims to consolidate existing literature on MVT cases and their indications, providing an organizational framework to com-prehend the current criteria for MVT.

Failure to close the abdomen after intestinal or multivisceral transplantation (Tx) remains a frequently occurring problem. Two attractive reconstruction methods, especially in large abdominal wall defects, are full-thickness abdominal wall vascularized composite allograft (AW-VCA) and nonvascularized rectus fascia (NVRF) Tx. This review compares surgical technique, immunology, integration, clinical experience, and indications of both techniques. In AW-VCA Tx, vascular anastomosis is required and the graft undergoes hypotrophy post-Tx. Furthermore, it has immunologic benefits and good clinical outcome. NVRF Tx is an easy technique without the need for vascular anastomosis. Moreover, a rapid integration and neovascularization occurs with excellent clinical outcome.

The traditional procedure for multivisceral transplant (MVT) is to transplant the stomach, pancreas, intestine, and liver en bloc. During surgery, the native spleen is routinely removed from the recipient, and it usually creates more space in the abdomen to insert the allogeneic graft. Thus, recipients often become asplenic after MVT. Considering all of the risks and benefits, we advocate that temporary transplant of the donor spleen could be the best option for MVT recipients; it could potentially reduce the rate of intestinal allograft rejection without increasing the risk for graft-versus-host disease.

Hirschsprung's disease is a dysmotility disease caused by lack of ganglion cells in the bowel wall that can affect varying lengths of the intestine. In extreme circumstances, there can be little remaining ganglionated bowel, and the patient becomes dependent on parental nutrition (PN) for survival. Intestinal transplant has been utilized to salvage these patients suffering terminal complications of PN. The question as to whether to reestablish intestinal continuity, and thus not require a stoma is vexed. However, data and experience would suggest this can be safely done with good functional results.

As we all acknowledge benefits of ostomies, they can come with significant morbidity, quality of life issues, and major complications, especially during reversal procedures. In recent years, we have started to observe that similar graft and patient survival can be achieved without ostomies in certain cases. This observation and practice adopted in a few large-volume transplant centers opened a new discussion about the necessity of ostomies in intestinal transplantation. There is still more time and randomized studies will be needed to better understand and analyze the risk/benefits of "No-ostomy" approach in intestinal transplantation.

Achieving feeding skills and food acceptance is a multi-layered process. In pediatric intestinal failure (PIF), oral feeding is important for feeding skills development, physiologic adaptation, quality of life and the prevention of eating disorders. In PIF, risk factors for feeding difficulties are common and early data suggests that feeding difficulties are prevalent. There is a unique paradigm for the feeding challenges in PIF. Conventional definitions of eating disorders have limited application in this context. A pediatric intestinal failure associated eating disorder (IFAED) definition that includes feeding/eating skills dysfunction, psychosocial dysfunction, and the influence on weaning nutrition support is proposed.

Infants and children with intestinal failure are at risk for pediatric feeding disorders, which challenge their oral feeding development. This article explores these challenges and offers several practical strategies that can be used by multidisciplinary care teams and at-home caregivers to help support the development of oral feeding in these children and eventually lead to their attaining enteral autonomy.

GASTROENTEROLOGY
CLINICS OF NORTH AMERICA

SERIES OF RELATED INTEREST

Clinics in Liver Disease
(https://www.liver.theclinics.com)
Gastrointestinal Endoscopy Clinics of North America
(https://www.giendo.theclinics.com)

THE CLINICS ARE AVAILABLE ONLINE!
Access your subscription at:
www.theclinics.com

Preface

Not Even a Ribbon for Intestinal Failure

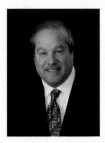

Alan L. Buchman, MD, MSPH
Editor

Possibly the most complex and heterogenous disease known to mankind, intestinal failure, had neither recognition nor a colored ribbon. There was no disease code in the *International Classification of Diseases, Tenth Revision, Clinical Modification* *(ICD-10CM)* or *ICD-11* for either intestinal failure or short bowel syndrome until October 1, 2023; still, there is no ribbon. All the primary color ribbons have been taken—even burgundy, cranberry, peach, and pink; light blue, dark blue, navy blue, and even Robin's egg blue; jade, light green, lime green, and mint green; cream, copper, and brown—yes brown: it's antitobacco and serves as a backup for colon cancer, I guess, in case they run out of whatever blue they are using. Brown runs in patients with intestinal failure and never seems to run out (literally). Why can't intestinal failure be awarded the brown ribbon? The failure of many organs seems to warrant a ribbon (pale blue for achalasia, emerald green for liver failure, green for renal failure, light blue for pulmonary failure, and blue for brain injury). Nothing though for intestinal failure—not even brown, which should be granted by rule of law.

Perhaps ribbons are really not the most appropriate; I'll submit that medals are probably much more appropriate for both the patients, their families, and their providers.

There are other forms of recognition, there is HPN (Home Parenteral Nutrition Awareness) Week, although no Hallmark card, and many diseases seem to get an entire month. Those patients with intestinal failure and their caregivers deserve much more than even a year.

Although most patients with intestinal failure do not require an intestinal transplant (kindly refer to the *Gastroenterology Clinics of North America* issue on Intestinal Rehabilitation, December, 2019), for those with potentially life-threatening complications of the disease, or perhaps even those with a high likelihood of a lifetime inability to work, inability to partake in many activities, and multiple hospitalizations for

---

Gastroenterol Clin N Am 53 (2024) xi–xii
https://doi.org/10.1016/j.gtc.2024.02.002
0889-8553/24/© 2024 Elsevier Inc. All rights reserved.

complications of intestinal failure, transplant can be lifesaving as well as life-changing. No longer hooked to a big IV in their chest or leg while they sleep. No longer getting up to use the bathroom several times a night. The intestinal transplant club is unique—the patients are unique as well as the providers, as heterogenous as both may be. Fewer than 100 such transplants are performed throughout the world annually, yet it is a very special club. Transplant and graft survival at one and five years now is consistent with that of those remaining on HPN. Patients that have successfully undergone intestinal, or multivisceral transplant, now are surviving 20 years or more, although overall a better understanding of chronic rejection is still required as longevity declines after 5 years.

Significant advancements in donor selection and preservation, surgical technique, and immunosuppression have led to remarkably improved outcomes. In this issue of *Gastroenterology Clinics of North America*, Drs Ladowski and Sudan address advances in organ preservation, while Dr Iyer and Dr Di Cocco and colleagues address the original indications as well as expanded indication for intestinal transplantation. More contemporary and advanced surgical techniques that have likely led to improved outcomes are covered by Drs Vianna, Muylle and colleagues, Matsumoto and Kato, and Dr Tekin and colleagues.

Despite these advances, successful intestinal transplantation may lead to problems not commonly envisioned. For example, a child that has been on nightly parenteral nutrition since birth and never really suckled or ate, doesn't even really know how to eat and must be trained to do so and thus be able to use their new bowel. Many of these children, their caregivers, and providers face these issues even prior to, or without transplant; potential countermeasures and therapy are addressed by Dr Boctor and colleagues as well as by Drs Hopkins and Merritt.

Intestinal failure may be the most complex disease that exists, and intestinal transplantation may be the most challenging transplant, no less disease therapy. This issue of *Gastroenterology Clinics of North America* is the first of a two-part series on intestinal transplantation. As such, it broaches just some of the significant issues facing these patients and providers but hopefully will enlighten readers and eventually improve care, either by primary providers or through referrals to the few specialized intestinal rehabilitation and transplant centers that exist in the world.

Alan L. Buchman, MD, MSPH
Intestinal Rehabilitation and Transplant Center
Department of Surgery/
UI Health University of Illinois at Chicago
840 South Wood Street
Suite 402 (MC958)
Chicago, IL 60612, USA

E-mail address:
buchman@uic.edu

Normothermic Preservation of the Intestinal Allograft

Joseph M. Ladowski, MD, PhD[a], Debra L. Sudan, MD[b],*

KEYWORDS

- Intestinal transplant ● Machine perfusion ● Normothermic machine perfusion
- Pig intestine ● Intestinal preservation

KEY POINTS

- The intestinal mucosa and allograft is particularly sensitive to ischemia and ischemia-reperfusion injury (IRI), providing unique challenges compared with other solid-organ allografts
- The sensitivity of the intestinal graft to IRI complicates the logistics of preserving the allograft
- Preservation of the intestinal graft for transplant has progressed from simple static cold storage to normothermic machine perfusion
- The current devices for machine perfusion of intestinal graft demonstrate good survival in a preclinical transplant model

HISTORY AND INDICATIONS

Originally introduced by Thomas Starzl in the 1960s, the first successful long-term intestinal transplant (IT) was reported to be completed in 1989.[1] IT is often combined with other abdominal organs—termed multivisceral transplantation. For the purposes of this review, we will focus on efforts related solely to IT and preservation.

IT is most often indicated for intestinal failure—inability of the gastrointestinal tract to absorb sufficient nutrients or water to maintain health.[2] Intestinal failure is a disease process with many causes—affecting both pediatric and adult patients. In children, it presents as short bowel due to many causes: surgical resection, necrotizing enterocolitis, intestinal atresia, and Hirschsprung disease. In adults, Crohn disease, mesenteric vascular occlusion, surgical complications, and trauma are the leading causes of intestinal failure.[3] The current initial management of intestinal failure is intestinal

Funded by: DOD. Grant number(s): PR181265P1; W81XWH-19-1-0677.
[a] Department of Surgery, Duke University Medical Center, Durham, NC, USA; [b] Division Chief of Abdominal Transplant in the Department of Surgery, Duke Transplant Center, Duke University School of Medicine, Durham, NC, USA
* Corresponding author. Department of Surgery, Duke University, 223 Hanes House, Durham, NC 22710.
E-mail address: debra.sudan@duke.edu

rehabilitation, which includes both medical (dietary changes, teduglutide, and total parenteral nutrition [TPN]) and surgical interventions (intestinal lengthening procedures and other autologous reconstruction techniques).[4-6] Unfortunately, these options are imperfect and TPN is associated with a significant infectious risk, catheter-related complications, and parenteral nutrition-associated liver disease.[7] For patients no longer able to be managed on TPN, IT represents the definitive treatment of intestinal failure.[8]

BENEFITS OF INTESTINAL TRANSPLANT

Successful IT is cost-effective compared with TPN within 1 to 3 years and associated with a significant increase in functional status, quality of life, and decreased anxiety.[9,10] Despite the advantages, IT is a technically challenging and labor-intensive operation with the risk for immunosuppression-related complications and not commonly performed. In 2022, only 82 IT were performed in the United States according to the United Network for Organ Sharing (**Fig. 1**). Additionally, long-term graft survival of IT seems to have stagnated and 10-year graft survival hovers around 30% to 40%.

CHALLENGES OF INTESTINAL TRANSPLANT

Unlike other solid organ transplants (eg, kidney, liver, and heart), intestinal transplantation is not limited per se by the availability of suitable organs but rather finding donors without risk for severe intestine injury from ischemic insult and graft preservation and the correct immunologic balance in the recipient between graft rejection and overwhelming infection.[7] This is partly due to the unique fact that the intestine is a hollow organ filled with bacteria particularly sensitive to donor brain death, ischemia-reperfusion injury (IRI), preservation-associated damage, and ischemia.[11-13] The IRI induced by procurement can lead to loss of epithelium at the villous tips and breakdown in the tight-junctions that are critical to the integrity and function of the cellular barrier. The tight-junctions and mucosal cell–cell connections are particularly important in IT because passive paracellular transfer of bacteria can lead to bacterial translocation and sepsis.[14-16] Furthermore, the intestinal epithelial cells have the complex task of food digestion and nutrient absorption, which can be impacted by the IRI.

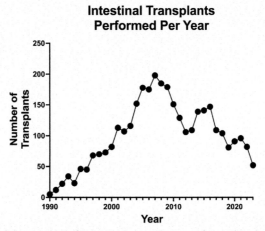

Fig. 1. Depiction of the number of intestinal transplants performed in the United States per year from 1990 to 2023 (data ongoing in 2023). (Data taken from the United Network for Organ Sharing webpage in Sept 2023.)

Additional challenges affecting the widespread application of IT are the logistical hurdles to IT. Only major academic institutions with highly skilled surgical teams can offer the operation because of the complexity of the procedure and postoperative care. This provides the first geographic constraint. Second, the current method of graft preservation further limits the field. There are no US Food and Drug Administration-approved commercially available devices for intestinal graft preservation and the standard of care is static cold storage (SCS). Unfortunately, the intestinal mucosa is exquisitely sensitive to hypoxia and within 1 hour of ischemia will show marked submucosal edema.[17] The intestine's susceptibility to hypoxia and IRI seems to be proportional to the length of the cold ischemia time.[18,19] As a result, transplant teams strive to perform the implantation within 6 to 10 hours of cold ischemia time, which limits the geographic radius of potential IT donors.[7]

SOLID ORGAN ALLOGRAFT PRESERVATION
History

The standard procurement and cold storage of donor organs means that solid organ transplantation requires a period of donor graft anoxia and cessation of perfusion. The resultant cellular hypoxia leads to an increase in anaerobic metabolism, deprivation of adenosine triphosphate, and accumulation of metabolic byproducts and reactive oxygen species. In the 1960s, it was theorized that cooling the donor graft would decrease the cellular metabolic activity and associated anoxic injury.[20] Before this time, it was common that experiments in normothermia and dynamic machine perfusion took place.[21] The target goal was 0°C to 4°C, which would result in a 95% reduction in cellular respiration and metabolism. In 1969, Collins and colleagues demonstrated successful preservation and transplantation of dog kidneys following 24 hours of SCS, and SCS became the gold standard for organ preservation.[22,23]

Although SCS remained the standard for many years, research in machine perfusion never stopped. One of the first hypothermic (goal temperature: 0°C–8°C) machine perfusion (HMP) models was developed by Dr Folkert Belzer, who used the device to perform the first HMP-preserved kidney transplant in 1968.[20,24] As the long-term outcomes improved and the number of successful transplants increased, there was an increasing need for a new donor organ source. Marginal or extended criteria donor (ECD) was a potential source. In the 1990s to 2000s, HMP saw an increase in popularity because transplant teams sought to use the ECD pool for renal transplantation.[21] One advantage to machine perfusion-preservation over SCS is the ability to simultaneously preserve, evaluate, and recondition the donor organ before transplantation.

Ultimately, the evidence demonstrated that HMP-preserved kidney grafts experienced less delayed graft function, and additional methods to further improve outcomes were pursued.[25] Normothermic machine perfusion (NMP), maintenance of the donor graft at 35°C to 38°C with the goal of maintaining metabolic activity and cellular viability, similarly experienced a resurgence in the 2000s. The goal is that by returning the graft to a physiologic state sooner, the donor organ can begin to repair and minimize the IRI that occurs. Multiple studies in heart and liver preservation demonstrate a benefit of NMP over SCS. Some of these benefits include but are not limited to donor pool expansion, prolonged ischemia time without loss of function, improved graft function, and decreased risk of rejection.[26–29] Furthermore, additional reports for human kidney HMP have reported superior outcomes with machine perfusion-preserved grafts compared with SCS.[29–31] Despite the advances in virtually all other solid organs, understanding the utility of machine perfusion (MP) in IT allografts is in its infancy.

Markers of Successful Preservation

Before discussing the advances in intestinal graft MP, it is important to first define how we identify intestinal mucosal injury and how to assess whether a preservation technique improves outcomes. The list detailed here is not exhaustive but represents some of the potential markers used to define success in intestinal graft preservation. The primary methods of measurement to be considered are the histologic, the cellular, and the biochemical.

Intestinal mucosa histologic evaluation

Tissue biopsy and histologic evaluation remain the gold standard for the identification of rejection and mucosal injury. The current standard for the classification of bowel IRI is the Park/Chiu score—a system ranging from 0 (normal mucosa) to 8 (transmural infarction).[32,33] This system owes its reliability to the sequential and predictable pattern in which intestinal mucosal injury occurs. Following an IRI resulting in edema, subepithelial clefts form at the villus tip, which is then followed by epithelia lifting from the lamina propria. This progresses to denuding of the villi from the lamina propria, and eventual loss of villi and mucosal infarction.[33] The majority of studies comparing intestinal IRI use this system, which provides some ability to compare results between studies/interventions (variation between pathologist readings aside). It is also important to recognize that species-specific differences may exist in the timing of ischemic injury. For example, when comparing pig to human intestines, human intestines typically demonstrate ischemia changes earlier compared with pig in an SCS model (8–14 vs 24 hours, respectively).[34]

Tissue markers

As discussed previously, the integrity of the intestinal mucosa and tight-junctions is particularly important to decrease bacterial translocation and rejection risk. As a result, the absence of markers associated with epithelial cell and tight-junction viability carry some prognostic capabilities. Although these markers require immunofluorescence staining and changes may not manifest immediately, there is an association between cellular health and presence of zona occludens - 1, claudin-3, and villin.[15,35–37] Additional markers to consider are the toll-like receptor (TLR) family, subsets of which are considered to be receptors for the metabolite ligands that mediate IRI.[38]

Biochemical markers

The goal of MP is to minimize cellular inflammation and apoptosis. As a result, perfusate levels of inflammatory cytokines (nuclear factor-κB, interleukin [IL]-2, IL-6, heat shock protein [HSP] 70, interferon-γ, and tumor necrosis factor alpha [TNFα]) may provide insight into the cellular trauma and graft dysfunction. Studies by Braun and colleagues demonstrate the IL-2, IL-6, HSP70, and interferon-γ (IFN-γ) seem to correlate with mRNA expression during intestinal IRI. The authors localize the expression of these cytokines to the intestinal endothelial, ganglion, and smooth muscle cells, providing valuable insight into how the vascular endothelium may respond to IRI that biopsy or tissue staining may not.[39]

ADVANCES IN INTESTINAL GRAFT MACHINE PERFUSION
Early Model Development (1960–70s)

The first description of an ex vivo perfusion of an intestinal graft segment is from 1967 in which Iijima and Salerno described a method of normothermic pulsatile perfusion of dog intestine for 5 hours followed by autotransplantation.[40] The authors define success in this study as "survival and function" of the excised, perfused, and transplanted intestinal graft. By this definition, they were able to achieve 2 week to 6-month survival in a series of dog ITs. The authors report grossly normal histology (this was before the formalization of the Park-Chiu score).

Concurrent research in intestinal graft preservation was taking place in the laboratory of Dr Richard Lillehei. Dr Lillehei first reported his research efforts in 1959, detailing the physiologic response of the dog intestine to ischemia and recognized the need for appropriate tissue preservation.[13] In 1971, Ruiz and colleagues detail an HMP system to perfuse dog intestine ex vivo for up to 48 hours. It is difficult to compare results of this experiment to the current era: success in this study was defined as "tissue viability" as studied by oxygen consumption, D-xylose absorption, and LDH production without transplantation.[19] The tissue was reportedly histologically normal at 12 hours of MP preservation, with changes in tissue quality noted with longer preservation times.

These early models provided scientific validation that an intestinal graft could be excised, perfused, and reimplanted while maintaining some degree of tissue integrity. Additionally, they laid the groundwork for further refinements in HMP and NMP.

Advancing the Model (1990s–2010s)

In 1998 Braun and colleagues provided the basis for the modern intestinal graft NMP device when they published an article detailing their development of an ex vivo intestinal graft perfusion device for pig intestines. The perfusion system described included a roller pump, perfusion chamber, hemofilter, blood pressure monitor, heater, oxygen blender, and oxygen/heat exchanger. The authors diagram how the SMA was perfused with whole blood, which was collected through the SMV or portal vein, entered into a blood reservoir, filtered, warmed, oxygenated, and perfused back into the SMA for recirculation.[41] Although the model was an overall success, reportedly, there seemed to be some tissue ischemia as evidenced by increasing arterial pressure and elevated lactate throughout the perfusion.

The field of MP in intestine allografts experienced a relative lull until 2014 when the Yale group published their results on the perfusion of intestines with a novel hypothermic intestinal perfusion unit (IPU) that included both a vascular and an intraluminal perfusion component.[42] Compared to an SCS control group, human intestines excised and perfused with the IPU demonstrated *improved* tissue histology as judged by the Park-Chiu score in 60% (3/5) of cases.[43] This represented one of the first times that MP was demonstrated to be potentially better than the current standard of SCS.

A group at the University of Cambridge expanded on these results and showed a possible role for NMP to *assess* the intestinal graft for injury and viability after reperfusion. The group obtained pig intestinal grafts from a slaughterhouse that were exposed to approximately 5 hours of CIT prior to reperfusion. There was a worse appearance in histology following reperfusion, exposing an important concept in MP of SCS graft: a period of machine perfusion might provide the opportunity to assess IRI in IT.[44] Mechanistically, the worsened histologic outcomes are likely due to the return of blood flow distributing the IRI metabolic products and other damage-associated metabolites to the entire intestinal mucosa and vascular endothelium. Without blood flow, it is likely that the IRI products of the intestinal segment are localized. A corollary to this situation is found with the traumatic "crush syndrome." Crush syndrome is the pathologic process that occurs following tissue reperfusion after a significant crush injury. This process is characterized not only by systemic electrolyte abnormalities and hypovolemic shock, but also local changes in the crushed tissue such as worsening skeletal muscle and microvascular injury *after* re-oxygenation.[45] The suspected mechanism is through reactive-oxygen species, as administration of a free radical scavenger can significantly ameliorate some of this injury.[46] Interestingly, the Cambridge group demonstrated no difference in tissue injury between leukocyte-depleted and whole blood perfusion. This finding suggests that IRI could be mediated by innate tissue factors rather than lymphocytic infiltration and activation.[44]

From Pump to Patient (2020s)

Significant advances had been made to the field of IT but, except for the early studies in a dog IT model, no reported literature detailed the results of an IT following MP (**Fig. 2**). Preliminary studies from our group at Duke University led to the hypothesis that a limitation of the Braun model was the inability to manage the metabolic issues in the small bowel, ultimately leading to graft acidosis, electrolyte disturbances, and poor regional perfusion. With this in mind, we developed and reported in 2022 an NMP device for the preservation of pig small intestine. The intestinal grafts preserved with this device were viable enough for transplantation.[48] We started with a model similar to the Braun model but multiple modifications were made to the preservation protocols and machinery.[41] The initial adjustments included (1) the addition of a perfusate dialysis component to address biochemical imbalances, (2) transition from 100% oxygen to carbogen in the perfusate to assist in perfusate pH regulation, (3) addition of vasodilatory medications to improve perfusion, and (d) infusion of nutrients. Following further refinements, a series of perfused intestinal grafts were deemed acceptable for transplantation and a total of 5 transplants were performed (**Fig. 3**).

Of the 5 orthotopic IT recipients, all 5 survived to the 48-hour study endpoint. Two of the 5 were found to have significant thrombotic complications in the pig cranial mesenteric artery and vein (the pig equivalent of the superior mesenteric artery and vein). This thrombosis resulted in ischemic bowel in the recipients, which was discovered on necropsy. The 3 remaining IT recipients without thrombotic complication were found to have grossly and histologically normal-appearing bowel at the time of necropsy. Since this time, an additional 2 pig ITs have been performed with our perfusion

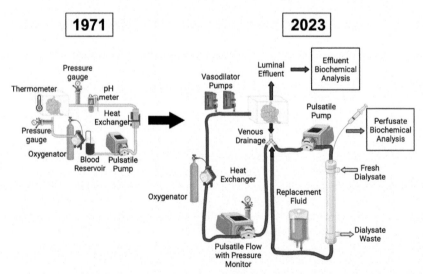

Fig. 2. A depiction of the advances made from the first described intestinal graft machine perfusion model (*left*) to the most recent NMP model (*right*) with multiple capabilities for perfusate and luminal effluent sampling, dialysis and metabolic control, dialysis, adjustments to perfusate biochemical composition, and vasodilatory medication titration. Created with BioRender.com.

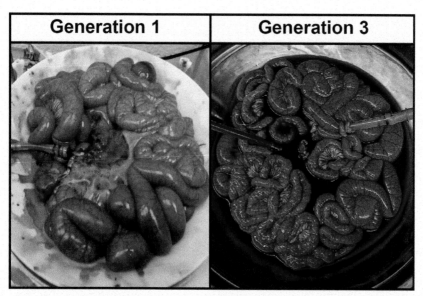

Fig. 3. Representative images reflecting the significant improvement in gross appearance and viability of the perfused intestinal graft between the first generation (*left-side image*) and the third-generation NMP (*right-side image*).

device with no evidence of reperfusion injury and appropriate postoperative bowel function.[47]

Subsequent study by Hou and colleagues further explored the potential advantages of HMP for the preservation of the intestine allograft as an alternative to NMP. This group compared the HMP preserved grafts to SCS using subsequent autotransplantation in 10 miniature pigs (n = 5 in each arm).[49] Both the SCS and HMP seemed grossly equivalent following 9 hours of CIT but histologically the HMP group demonstrated less edema and villous trauma than the SCS group. Furthermore, the return of blood flow to the SCS graft intraoperatively revealed signs of tissue injury (lack of peristalsis and dark/swollen tissue). However, the HMP-preserved intestine seemed rosy in color with good peristaltic movement and superior histologic scores at the time of reperfusion.

Postoperatively, 1 of the 5 (20%) SCS-preserved IT recipients survived to end of study (7 days). The other pigs in the SCS arm demonstrated concerning physical examination features such as abdominal distension and infrequent stool. The eventual necropsy findings were consistent with intestinal necrosis and severe abdominal infection.

The HMP-preserved intestine was superior to the SCS-preserved in all studied ways following reperfusion at the time of transplantation: microcirculation as measured by laser Doppler, histologic changes as determined by electron microscopy, and survival. The recipients of the HMP preserved intestinal segment demonstrated return of bowel function, no bloody stool, and 100% survival (n = 5) to 7 days. This study also examined potential biomarkers that might be used to assess intestine preservation including, immunofluorescence of tight junction proteins (occludin and ZO-1), inflammatory cytokine changes (demonstrated decreased IL-1, IL-6, IFN-γ, TNF-α, TLR4, and NFkB in HMP preserved grafts), and decreased caspase 3 activity (representing apoptotic activity). Additionally, at 1-hour postreperfusion in transplant recipients, sera levels of IL-1b, IL-6, IL-10, IFN-γ, and TNF-α were all significantly better in the HMP-preserved versus SCS-preserved intestine allografts.[49]

FUTURE OF INTESTINAL TRANSPLANT

Recent advances made with MP preservation of IT grafts suggest an increasing optimism in the field. The path forward has been partially laid by the examples set in other solid organ allografts. It seems plausible that successful intestinal graft MP will decrease IRI, reduce logistical barriers to transplant (eg, the travel radius for donor grafts), and improve outcomes by decreasing early infections due to better mucosal and epithelial barrier integrity, as well as, potentially decreasing rejection rates due to less early inflammatory response to the graft. Furthermore, as outcomes improve, a compelling case could be made that IT should be initiated earlier in the intestinal rehabilitation process.

Enthusiasm for IT must be tempered by the recognition that the field of MP of the intestine allograft is still in its infancy. The next logical step is further research in the development of an MP device to be used in clinical trials for human application. Additionally, although the focus of this review has been on the advancements in preservation, MP also allows for the opportunity to evaluate intestinal grafts before implantation. Although some of the potential metrics to assess viability of an intestine graft have been discussed here: (A) gross tissue appearance; (B) biopsy samples demonstrating histologic changes as well as IF changes in ZO-1, occludin, villin; and (C) organ perfusate levels of metabolic and apoptotic activity, the optimal markers remain to be defined. As intestinal MP volume increases experimentally and eventually clinically, there will likely be a further role for the evaluation of these markers and correlations between biomarker level and graft function.

As best shown in ex vivo donor lung perfusion, MP provides the opportunity to expand the donor pool by reconditioning and thereby improving the performance and function of a graft. One example in lung transplant comes from documented reports of treating bacteria laden donor lungs with antibiotic perfusion to treat the infection pretransplant.[50] Additional examples of preoperative reconditioning include the attenuation of the lung IRI with direct cytokine removal, N-acetyl cysteine, or steroids.[51–54] It is not difficult to imagine the opportunity to recondition the intestine allograft and expand the current intestine donor pool. Perhaps, this could be performed by an intraluminal bowel prep or administration of nutrients or medications to assist with the restoration of epithelial and tight junction integrity in a donor that has suffered prolonged hypotension or cardiac arrest.[50] Finally, the ability to perform gene therapy during the perfusion process has been discussed expertly elsewhere and the door is open for these avenues as well.[55]

SUMMARY

MP and NMP have a bright future for IT—the models have progressed from a simple pulsatile flow device to a complete normothermic perfusion system. Experimentally, we have demonstrated reproducible superior outcomes after transplantation of NMP intestine allografts compared with SCS and others have demonstrated similar superior outcomes using HMP compared with SCS. Translation of these findings to clinical utility is the next step. As the technology and research advances, new opportunities for improvement will present and the scope of IT will likely broaden to include earlier intervention, new indications, and new procedures. It is undoubtable that MP will be a key component of that progress.

CLINICS CARE POINTS

- There have been significant advances in the field of NMP of intestinal grafts
- Caution is recommended when comparing results of studies from pig to human
- It is likely that machine perfusion of intestinal grafts will be ready for clinical application in the coming years

DISCLOSURE

The authors report no conflicts of interest pertaining to this publication. J.M. Ladowski is supported by NIH, United States grant 1F32AI174651-01A1 and the American Society of Transplant Surgeons, United States Jon Fryer Resident Scientist Scholarship. D.L. Sudan is supported by the Department of Defense, United States W81XWH-19-1-0676, W81XWH-19-1-0677.

REFERENCES

1. Grant D, Wall W, Mimeault R, et al. Successful small-bowel/liver transplantation. Lancet 1990;335:181–4.
2. Allan P, Lal S. Intestinal failure: a review. F1000Res 2018;7:85.
3. Grant D, Abu-Elmagd K, Mazariegos G, et al. Intestinal Transplant Registry Report: Global Activity and Trends. AJT 2015;15:210–9.
4. Modi BP, Langer M, Ching YA, et al. Improved survival in a multidisciplinary short bowel syndrome program. J Pediatr Surg 2008;43:20–4.
5. Harpain F, Schlager L, Hütterer E, et al. Teduglutide in short bowel syndrome patients: A way back to normal life? JPEN - J Parenter Enter Nutr 2022;46:300–9.
6. Burness CB, McCormack P L Teduglutide. A Review of its Use in the Treatment of Patients with Short Bowel Syndrome. Drugs 2013;73:935–47.
7. Weissenbacher A, Vrakas G, Nasralla D, et al. The future of organ perfusion and re-conditioning. Transpl Int 2019;32:586–97.
8. Rege A, Sudan D. Intestinal transplantation. Best Pract Res Clin Gastroenterol 2016;30:319–35.
9. Holdaway L, Loo L, Smith A, et al. Intestinal Transplant Improves Quality of Life for Patients with Chronic Intestinal Failure. Transplantation 2017;101:S94.
10. Bharadwaj S, Tandon P, Gohel TD, et al. Current status of intestinal and multivisceral transplantation. Gastroenterol Rep (Oxf) 2017;5:20–8.
11. Koudstaal LG, 't Hart NA, Ploeg RJ, et al. Inflammation and structural changes in donor intestine and liver after brain death induction. Eur J Gastroenterol Hepatol 2005;17:A44.
12. Koudstaal LG, t Hart NA, van den Berg A, et al. Brain death causes structural and inflammatory changes in donor intestine. Transplant Proc 2005;37:448–9.
13. Lillehei RC, Goott B, Miller FA. The physiological response of the small bowel of the dog to ischemia including prolonged in vitro preservation of the bowel with successful replacement and survival. Ann Surg 1959;150:543–60.
14. Berg RD. Bacterial translocation from the gastrointestinal tract. Adv Exp Med Biol 1999;473:11–30.
15. Jiang Y, Guo C, Zhang D, et al. The Altered Tight Junctions: An Important Gateway of Bacterial Translocation in Cachexia Patients with Advanced Gastric Cancer. J Interferon Cytokine Res 2014;34:518–25.

16. Zeitouni NE, Chotikatum S, von Köckritz-Blickwede M, et al. The impact of hypoxia on intestinal epithelial cell functions: consequences for invasion by bacterial pathogens. Molecular and Cellular Pediatrics 2016;3:14.

17. Tesi RJ, Jaffe BM, McBride V, et al. Histopathologic changes in human small intestine during storage in viaspan organ preservation solution. Arch Pathol Lab Med 1997;121:714–8.

18. Takeyoshi I, Zhang S, Nomoto M, et al. Mucosal damage and recovery of the intestine after prolonged preservation and transplantation in dogs. Transplantation 2001;71:1–7.

19. Ruiz OJ, Schultz LS, Hendrickx J, et al. Isolated intestinal perfusion:: a method for assessing preservation methods and viability before transplantation. Am Soc Artif Intern Organs J 1971;17:42.

20. Belzer FolkertO, Ashby BS, Dunphy JE. 24-hour and 72-hour preservation of canine kidneys. Lancet 1967;290:536–9.

21. Jing L, Yao L, Zhao M, et al. Organ preservation: from the past to the future. Acta Pharmacol Sin 2018;39:845–57.

22. Collins GM, Bravo-Shugarman M, Terasaki PI. Kidney preservation for transportation: Initial Perfusion and 30 Hours' Ice Storage. Lancet 1969;294:1219–22.

23. Collins GM, Bravo-Shugarman M, Terasaki PI, et al. Kidney Preservation for Transportation: IV. Eight-Thousand-Mile International Air Transport1. Aust N Z J Surg 1970;40:195–7.

24. Belzer FO, Ashby BS, Gulyassy PF, et al. Successful seventeen-hour preservation and transplantation of human-cadaver kidney. N Engl J Med 1968;278:608–10.

25. Henry SD, Guarrera JV. Protective effects of hypothermic ex vivo perfusion on ischemia/reperfusion injury and transplant outcomes. Transplant Rev 2012;26:163–75.

26. Koerner MM, Ghodsizad A, Schulz U, et al. Normothermic ex vivo allograft blood perfusion in clinical heart transplantation. Heart Surg Forum 2014;17:E141–5.

27. Ardehali A, Esmailian F, Deng M, et al. Ex-vivo perfusion of donor hearts for human heart transplantation (PROCEED II): a prospective, open-label, multicentre, randomised non-inferiority trial. Lancet 2015;385:2577–84.

28. Schroder JN, Patel CB, DeVore AD, et al. Transplantation Outcomes with Donor Hearts after Circulatory Death. N Engl J Med 2023;388:2121–31.

29. van Rijn R, Schurink IJ, de Vries Y, et al. Hypothermic Machine Perfusion in Liver Transplantation — A Randomized Trial. N Engl J Med 2021;384:1391–401.

30. Nicholson ML, Hosgood SA. Renal Transplantation After Ex Vivo Normothermic Perfusion: The First Clinical Study. Am J Transplant 2013;13:1246–52.

31. Hosgood SA, Callaghan CJ, Wilson CH, et al. Normothermic machine perfusion versus static cold storage in donation after circulatory death kidney transplantation: a randomized controlled trial. Nat Med 2023;29:1511–9.

32. Chiu CJ, McArdle AH, Brown R, et al. Intestinal mucosal lesion in low-flow states. I. A morphological, hemodynamic, and metabolic reappraisal. Arch Surg 1970;101:478–83.

33. Park PO, Haglund U, Bulkley GB, et al. The sequence of development of intestinal tissue injury after strangulation ischemia and reperfusion. Surgery 1990;107:574–80.

34. Søfteland JM, Casselbrant A, Biglarnia AR, et al. Intestinal Preservation Injury: A Comparison Between Rat, Porcine and Human Intestines. Int J Mol Sci 2019;20:3135.

35. Kuo W-T, Zuo L, Odenwald MA, et al. The Tight Junction Protein ZO-1 Is Dispensable for Barrier Function but Critical for Effective Mucosal Repair. Gastroenterology 2021;161:1924–39.

36. Barmeyer C, Schulzke JD, Fromm M. Claudin-related intestinal diseases. Semin Cell Dev Biol 2015;42:30–8.

37. Wang Y, Srinivasan K, Siddiqui MR, et al. A novel role for villin in intestinal epithelial cell survival and homeostasis. J Biol Chem 2008;283:9454–64.

38. Sukhotnik I, Ben Shahar Y, Halabi S, et al. Effect of N-Acetylserotonin on TLR-4 and MyD88 Expression during Intestinal Ischemia-Reperfusion in a Rat Model. Eur J Pediatr Surg 2019;29:188–95.

39. Braun F, Hosseini M, Wieland E, et al. Kinetics and localization of interleukin-2, interleukin-6, heat shock protein 70, and interferon gamma during intestinal-rerfusion injury. Transplant Proc 2004;36:267–9.

40. Iijima K, Salerno RA. Survival of small intestine following excision, perfusion and autotransplantation. Ann Surg 1967;166:968–75.

41. Braun F, Schütz E, Laabs S, et al. Development of a porcine small bowel ex vivo perfusion model. Transplant Proc 1998;30:2613–5.

42. Narayan RR, Pancer NE, Loeb BW, et al. A novel device to preserve intestinal tissue ex-vivo by cold peristaltic perfusion. Annu Int Conf IEEE Eng Med Biol Soc 2014;3118–21.

43. Muñoz-Abraham AS, Patrón-Lozano R, Narayan RR, et al. Extracorporeal Hypothermic Perfusion Device for Intestinal Graft Preservation to Decrease Ischemic Injury During Transportation. J Gastrointest Surg 2016;20:313–21.

44. Hamed MO, Barlow AD, Dolezalova N, et al. Ex vivo normothermic perfusion of isolated segmental porcine bowel: a novel functional model of the small intestine. BJS Open 2021;5:zrab009.

45. Odeh M. The Role of Reperfusion-Induced Injury in the Pathogenesis of the Crush Syndrome. N Engl J Med 1991;324:1417–22.

46. Walker PM, Lindsay TF, Labbe R, et al. Salvage of skeletal muscle with free radical scavengers. J Vasc Surg 1987;5:68–75.

47. Ludwig EK, Abraham N, Schaaf CR, et al. Comparison of the effects of normothermic machine perfusion and cold storage preservation on porcine intestinal allograft regenerative potential and viability. Am J Transplant 2023; S1600-6135(23)00828-6..

48. Abraham N, Ludwig EK, Schaaf CR, et al. Orthotopic Transplantation of the Full-length Porcine Intestine After Normothermic Machine Perfusion. Transplantation Direct 2022;8:e1390.

49. Hou W, Yang S, Lu J, et al. Hypothermic machine perfusion alleviates ischemia-reperfusion injury of intestinal transplantation in pigs. Front Immunol 2023;14.

50. Nakajima D, Cypel M, Bonato R, et al. Ex Vivo Perfusion Treatment of Infection in Human Donor Lungs. Am J Transplant 2016;16:1229–37.

51. Geudens N, Wuyts WA, Rega FR, et al. N-acetyl cysteine attenuates the inflammatory response in warm ischemic pig lungs. J Surg Res 2008;146:177–83.

52. Martens A, Boada M, Vanaudenaerde BM, et al. Steroids can reduce warm ischemic reperfusion injury in a porcine donation after circulatory death model with ex vivo lung perfusion evaluation. Transpl Int 2016;29:1237–46.

53. Boffini M, Marro M, Simonato E, et al. Cytokines Removal During Ex-Vivo Lung Perfusion: Initial Clinical Experience. Transpl Int 2023;36:10777.

54. Kakishita T, Oto T, Hori S, et al. Suppression of inflammatory cytokines during ex vivo lung perfusion with an adsorbent membrane. Ann Thorac Surg 2010; 89:1773–9.

55. Pavan-Guimaraes J, Martins PN. Modifying organs with gene therapy and gene modulation in the age of machine perfusion. Curr Opin Organ Transplant 2022; 27:474–80.

Indications for Intestinal Transplantation

Kishore R. Iyer, MBBS, FRCS (Eng)

KEYWORDS

- Intestine • Transplant • Indications • Pre-emptive

KEY POINTS

- Intestine failure outcomes have improved with improvements in multidisciplinary care provided by expert intestinal rehabilitation programs.
- There have been parallel improvements in intestinal transplant outcomes.
- Late referrals for intestinal transplant are a serious ongoing problem, impacting both waitlist mortality and post-transplant outcomes.
- The author proposes a conceptual framework for a more collaborative approach that allows earlier identification of patients at risk for PN failure who should be referred earlier for intestinal transplant evaluation.

INTRODUCTION

Chronic intestinal failure (CIF) is a devastating condition where individuals cannot absorb nutrients and water required to meet their needs. Patients with CIF are dependent on parenteral nutrition (PN) administered intravenously to provide carbohydrates, protein, fat with water, electrolytes, trace elements, and vitamins to maintain health.[1–4] PN is administered over many hours each day to the patient and requires a long-term, indwelling central venous catheter (CVC).[5,6] Patients are tethered to an infusion pump and if they infuse at night, are unable to enjoy an uninterrupted night's sleep due to the various pump alarms and the increased frequency of urination from intravenous infusion. This has a significantly adverse impact on patient quality of life (QOL).[7–10] While PN is lifesaving in CIF, long-term PN is complicated by severe morbidities, including episodes of dehydration, CVC-related blood stream infections (CRBSIs) with associated sepsis, and intestinal failure-associated liver disease (IFALD), all leading to increased hospitalizations and cost.[11–20] Hospitalizations for patients with CIF who have short bowel syndrome (SBS) increased by 55%, from 4037 hospitalizations in 2005 to 6265 hospitalizations in 2014, due to complications of fluid and electrolyte abnormalities (52.5%), CRBSI with associated sepsis (41.4%), and malnutrition (40.1%).

Intestinal Rehabilitation & Transplant Program, Icahn School of Medicine at Mount Sinai and Mount Sinai Hospital, One Gustave Levy Place, Box 1104, New York 10029, USA
E-mail address: kishore.iyer@mountsinai.org

Gastroenterol Clin N Am 53 (2024) 233–244
https://doi.org/10.1016/j.gtc.2024.02.001
0889-8553/24/© 2024 Elsevier Inc. All rights reserved.

These data underscore the magnitude and complexity of CIF and the substantial utilization of health care resources needed for each patient with CIF.[19] A recently approved drug (teduglutide, glucagon-like-peptide-2 (GLP-2)) for SBS-related intestinal failure allows some patients to wean off PN but at considerable cost, estimated at $300,000 per year and with potential for significant side effects, including growth of colonic polyps and cancers.[21–24] The only potentially definitive cure for CIF is intestinal transplantation (ITX), which allows patients who are failing PN due to complications the prospect of eating and drinking normally and being free of PN. At costs estimated to exceed $1 million per transplant and the potential severe morbidity and even mortality of lifelong immunosuppression and its attendant life-threatening complications, ITX is reserved for patients with life-threatening complications of PN.[25]

CENTERS FOR MEDICARE AND MEDICAID SERVICES CRITERIA FOR INTESTINAL TRANSPLANT CONSIDERATION

In 2002, the Centers for Medicare and Medicaid Services (CMS) approved ITX for adult patients as no longer being experimental and approved pediatric ITX shortly thereafter.[25,26] In determining criteria for ITX, Medicare noted the excellent outcomes achieved by patients with CIF on home PN (HPN) with 1 year survival upward of 90% and 4 year survival being of the order of 80% to 85%.[26–29] Taking into account the relatively poor outcomes for ITX hitherto reported, Medicare established criteria for ITX that firmly recognized PN as the standard of care for patients with CIF and expressly reserved ITX for patients with permanent CIF who were also exhibiting signs of PN failure in the form of life-threatening complications of PN. Thus, the Medicare criteria for ITX could be summarized as the presence of irreversible CIF, which, for practical purposes, is irreversible PN-dependency and the onset of PN-related complications, most frequently IFALD or catheter-related complications including recurrent life-threatening sepsis, a single episode of fungal sepsis or metastatic infections such as endocarditis or osteomyelitis, and loss of central venous access due to central venous stenosis or thrombosis. Medicare also recognized the occurrence of less frequent PN complications such as metabolic abnormalities related to PN or unmanageable fluid and electrolyte abnormalities.[26,27] It is important to note that CMS proposed these criteria as broad criteria for consideration of ITX rather than their occurrence in some manner, mandating the performance of ITX.

The Medicare criteria for ITX have been flawed and problematic from their very inception for several reasons. Medicare erroneously concluded that irrespective of residual gastrointestinal anatomy or underlying disease, all patients with CIF on PN had the same potential long-term survival.[28,29] By selecting only those patients who were experiencing potentially life-threatening PN-related complications for ITX, patients referred for ITX had a theoretic zero chance of survival on continued PN, yet ITX outcomes in this higher risk cohort of patients with CIF were still compared to the best outcomes reported for patients with CIF on PN. The time taken from decision to refer a pateint for ITX evaluation to the date of ITX is variable and often prolonged. Several factors can contribute to this including the medical complexity of the pateint, the need to travel long distances to a referral center and prolonged waiting times after being placed on the wait-list for an approproate donor. Predictably then, delays in referral for ITX evaluation can lead to many patients with CIF needing cimultaneous liver replacement at the time of ITX, with a much higher mortality on the waiting list.[30,31] Thus, continued poor outcomes for ITX which were at least in part related to ITX being performed on only very high-risk patients with CIF, still being compared to the best outcomes for patients with CIF on PN perpetuated the self-fulfilling prophesy that

ITX was not ready for prime time and had to be reserved only for those patients with CIF in whom continued PN is impossible or dangerous. An additional lost opportunity occurred from failure to take into account any QOL considerations in decision-making retiming of ITX.

EVOLVING INDICATIONS FOR INTESTINAL TRANSPLANTATION

The last decade has seen recognition of the improving outcomes for ITX and the need for the indications to evolve with improvements in understanding and outcomes of ITX.[31-35] Examples of such indications include a nonreconstructible gastrointestinal tract on the basis of complex enteroatmospheric fistulae that have failed conservative surgical attempts, nonresectable soft tissue tumors at the root of the mesentery especially locally aggressive desmoid tumors occurring in the setting of familial adenomatous polyposis or multicystic lymphangiomas,[36-39] and not surprisingly, patients who had had a prior failed intestinal transplant with loss of allograft due to technical causes, severe acute rejection, or chronic rejection. For the first time also, a consideration of "patient choice" that is, patients not accepting a life on PN but preferring to pursue ITX was regarded as an acceptable indication for ITX. Pironi and colleagues looked at the epidemiology of ITX candidacy among European centers.[40] Approximately 12% of adult candidates and pediatric candidates were deemed to be candidates for ITX on the basis of high morbidity CIF or HPN refusal.[40,41]

A larger prospective 5 year study compared 389 noncandidates for ITX who had neither indication nor contraindications for ITX, with 156 candidates for ITX.[42] Candidacy for ITX was determined by the standard Medicare criteria for ITX.[42] The investigators observed that patients who were clinically stable on HPN enjoyed greater survival probability than ITX recipients.[42] While early mortality on HPN was primarily driven by the underlying disease, mortality in longer term survivors on HPN was related to complications of PN. Patients with IFALD and inoperable intra-abdominal desmoid tumors appeared to have survival advantage with earlier ITX.[42] This study raised some methodological concerns. The study excluded 271 patients on HPN who had contraindications for ITX based on high risk of death after ITX, ignoring the possibility that of the patients with organ failure in this cohort, timelier referral may have allowed some patients to survive following earlier ITX. This study, like most comparisons of survival of patients with CIF on HPN versus ITX, ignores the fact that the comparisons are not of 2 fundamentally comparable cohorts with equivalent survival potential, since the patients being referred for ITX due to HPN complications were already self-selected to do poorly on continued HPN. It is noteworthy that of 9 patients in this series who underwent ITX as a life-saving measure for PN-related complications, primarily IFALD, 6 of the 9 candidates required simultaneous liver replacement, indicating late referral.[42]

Kaufman and colleagues acknowledged in a recent consensus study that while QOL by itself could not constitute an indication for transplant given the lifelong morbidity and potential mortality risk from immunosuppression, QOL was excellent among survivors of ITX and QOL could hence be used as one additional consideration in the decision to proceed with ITX.[43] The investigators also noted the wait-list dynamics and a small but real mortality on the waiting list for patients awaiting ITX, especially if also awaiting simultaneous liver replacement.[31,44,45]

Pironi and colleagues proposed more "liberalized" indications for ITX based on the consensus study written by Kauffman and colleagues[43,46]; however, the plea for early referral for ITX was offset by the use of laboratory and clinical criteria for IFALD that reflect advanced liver disease with portal hypertension that inevitably would require simultaneous liver replacement at the time of ITX.[46] In discussing improved QOL post-ITX among adult patients, the investigators cautiously noted that individual expert centers reported excellent survival after isolated ITX and hence agreed that individual patients reporting poor QOL on HPN could be considered for pre-emptive ITX before the onset of complications. The concern raised by inferior graft survival compared to patient survival, post-ITX is, in our view irrelevant, since at worst, it returns the patient to a life on PN, the baseline state.

A clear but important indication for multivisceral transplant in the absence of intestinal failure arises in patients with confluent portomesenteric venous thrombosis and refractory portal hypertension who are not candidates for any kind of portosystemic shunt surgery or even salvage percutaneous or devascularization procedures and cannot received isolated liver transplant for technical reasons, due to the lack of suitable portal venous inflow. These patients require resection and removal of the involved abdominal organs with replacement of a multivisceral cluster allograft.[47,48] These transplants are still performed in small numbers in potentially very sick patients, and outcomes remain guarded, particularly when early access to suitable organs is impossible.[30] Recent changes in organ allocation for this uniquely challenging cohort of patients may allow improved outcomes in this very sick cohort. It should be noted in this context that ITX is best viewed as occurring in a composite graft; the 3 commonest types of ITX are shown in (**Fig. 1**).

REVISED PEDIATRIC INDICATIONS FOR INTESTINAL TRANSPLANTATION

Burghardt and colleagues from the Hospital for Sick Children, Toronto, evaluated the old 2001 intestinal listing criteria proposed by Kaufman and colleagues.[49,50] The 2001 criteria consisting of advanced cholestasis, loss of at least half central venous access sites, occurrence of 2 or more catheter-related sepsis episodes, and ultrashort bowel were compared in children with CIF in a prior era (1998–2005, $n = 99$) to a more contemporary era (2006–2012, $n = 91$). Two of the 2001 criteria had poor predictive value in the modern era—advanced cholestasis had a positive predictive value (PPV) of 64% in the old era and only 40% in the modern era, with sensitivity dropping from 84% to 65%, respectively. Similarly, ultrashort bowel, which had a PPV of 100% in the old era, had a PPV of only 9% in the modern era with a sensitivity of 105% and 4%, respectively. In contrast, 3 newly proposed criteria—(1) 2 or more Intensive Care Unit (ICU) admissions, (2) persistent bilirubin greater than 75 mmol/L (>4.4 mg/dL), and (3) loss of greater than 3 central venous access sites—had a high predictive value.[49]

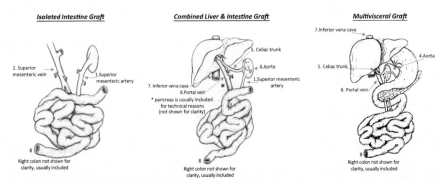

Fig. 1. Small bowel transplant occurs in composite visceral grafts.

Interestingly, the investigators estimated a greater than 98% need for ITX if 2 of the 3 criteria were met.[50]

Roberts and colleagues looked at a large international cohort of children (n = 443 children diagnosed with CIF between 2010 and 2015), with a primary outcome of death or ITX, in an attempt to validate the Toronto listing criteria proposed by Burghardt and colleagues.[50,51] The validated criteria had a high predictive value of death/IT and ≥ 2 ICU admissions ($P \geq$ .00001, OR 10.2, 95% CI 4.0–25.6; persistent conjugated hyperbilirubinemia, $P <$ .0001, OR 8.2, 95% CI 4.8–13.9; and loss of ≥ 3 central venous access sites, $P =$ .0003, OR 5.7, 95% CI 2.2–14.7). As the investigators point out, there is a clear case to refine modern pediatric listing criteria for ITX based on the Toronto listing criteria.[51]

INDICATIONS FOR INTESTINAL RETRANSPLANTATION

ITX is a high-risk endeavor with small but real risk of graft loss. Early graft loss might occur due to technical reasons such as graft ischemia or irreversible severe acute rejection.[52] However, as with all organ transplants, with increasing long-term survival of ITX recipients, it is clear that late graft loss due to chronic allograft enteropathy or chronic rejection occurs in 7% to 10% of cases.[33] In this situation, careful management of immunosuppression with retransplantation in well-selected recipients can allow successful long-term patient survival with a functioning second allograft.[53,54] Our own experience is in line with others from larger, more experienced centers suggesting that in well-selected recipients, carefully planned ITX retransplantation allows outcomes that approach those of first-time ITX. The need to manage careful immunosuppression during the transition and induction of the second allograft, managing risks of sepsis and allosensitization with development of preformed antibodies and technical factors including planning the vascular reconstruction for the second graft, become important considerations that impact survival.[53,54]

NEED FOR A MORE NUANCED APPROACH

The earliest multidisciplinary (multi-D) intestinal rehabilitation programs (IRPs) in the early part of this century were often extensions of leading ITX programs, for example, in Omaha, Nebraska, and Pittsburgh, Pennsylvania. The widespread adoption of multi-D IRPs since represents a paradigm shift in care of patients with CIF and has led to improved outcomes in CIF care, now being recognized as the means to deliver best outcomes for CIF.[55–57] It is important to emphasize that individual clinicians and HPN programs predating these IRPs were providing excellent care to patients with CIF, even if the value of multi-D care had not been established. Pari passu with the development of IRPs, there has been an explosion in knowledge in ITX across technical, immunologic, infectious, and QOL domains, all leading to improved outcomes following ITX. There has been an inescapable schism between the proponents of intestinal rehabilitation and the intestinal transplant community with a failure to acknowledge and recognize the complementary roles that these approaches may play and to treat them almost as mutually exclusive and even competing therapies. This has led to charges of early and inappropriate transplants on the one hand versus delayed and even doomed referrals on the other. The reconfiguration of the international intestinal transplant association and its formal designation as the International Intestinal Rehabilitation and Transplant Association is a welcome step in the right direction that might allow cooler minds to evaluate the limited data available and adopt more nuanced approaches to referral of patients with CIF to ITX centers in more timely manner and to recognize opportunities for intestinal rehabilitation which might hitherto have been missed. There are clues to how such an approach might be adopted in early work from Messing and colleagues that showed that adult patients with SBS who had about 100 cm of residual bowel had excellent prospects for intestinal rehabilitation and to achieve enduring freedom from PN.[58] In contrast, patients with less than 50 cm of residual small bowel had a high likelihood of permanent PN dependence without the prospect of achieving enteral autonomy and a correspondingly poor long-term survival.[58] Amiot and colleagues from the same group showed that 5 year survival in patients with "permanent" intestinal failure was about 60% at 5 years and indeed quite far from the 85% to 90% 5 year survival that was viewed as the achievable outcome among all patients on PN when ITX indications were codified.[59] A more recent study by Pironi and colleagues looked at 1 year survival among a large cohort (n = 2194 patients from 51 centers) and showed that 1 year survival on PN strongly correlated with both the volume and type of nutritional support (intravenous fluids alone or type and amount of macronutrients) in PN, serving as potential surrogates for severity of CIF.[60] In a large single-center study of 313 children with CIF, Fullerton and colleagues showed that transplant-free survival was excellent in children who achieved enteral autonomy versus children who did not achieve enteral autonomy, being 98.5% versus 94.1% at 1 year and 95.5% versus 86.7% at 5 years (P = .29).[61] A larger multicenter, multinational pediatric study published just a year prior, similarly showed that the incidence of enteral autonomy was only 53% at the 6 year mark.[62]

PROPOSED "RATIONAL" APPROACH

When PN-dependency is unequivocally irreversible, the traditional criteria of loss of 3 or more vascular access sites or end-stage liver disease, far from being simply indications for ITX, represent stigmata of late referral for ITX. In this context, it is important to recognize that the patient who presents for consideration of ITX with a translumbar IVC catheter or a transhepatic catheter is a high-risk ITX candidate for reasons that have everything to do with HPN care and sometimes misguided attempts at intestinal rehabilitation and very little to do with ITX-related events. Other examples abound for the impact of late referral on ITX outcomes. The vast subset of patients with irreversible IF referred for ITX with liver disease to the extent that they require simultaneous liver replacement (with a much higher risk of mortality on the waiting list) or the patients with multiple, recurrent catheter-related infections who become highly sensitized, by developing preformed antibodies against population antigens are higher risk ITX candidates at risk of poorer ITX outcomes on the basis of late referral.

The data in the previous section provide a clue to developing a better approach to identifying patients early for transplant. Patients with CIF who have the potential to achieve freedom from PN should be managed within an aggressive and dedicated multi-D IRP with a focus on achieving enteral autonomy and freedom from PN. If this is safely and robustly achieved there should be no further consideration for ITX. If, however, PN-dependency appears irreversible on initial assessment based on underlying disease (eg, idiopathic pseudo-obstruction or global intestinal dysmotility) or accurate understanding of gastrointestinal anatomy or appears irreversible on careful reassessments when intestinal rehabilitation attempts fail, then an early conversation and even evaluation for ITX is appropriate. This is underpinned by clear understanding and agreement that consideration or evaluation for ITX is only the first step in multi-D evaluation and does not commit either the patient or the care provider team to ITX. Such an approach of expanding the multi-D intestinal rehabilitation team to include the in-house intestinal transplant

team or the regional ITX center will ensure the best individualized plan of care for every patient with CIF and hopefully ensure that every patient with CIF gets the best opportunity to achieve freedom from PN. If attempts at intestinal rehabilitation are not proceeding well and ITX appears likely, there is every opportunity to do it early and in timely manner.

PRE-EMPTIVE INTESTINAL TRANSPLANTATION

As outcomes of intestinal rehabilitation continue to improve, especially with teduglutide joining the armamentarium of available multimodality therapies, the case for "pre-emptive" intestinal transplant might appear ever more challenging. However, "pre-emptive" in this context should be viewed as "before the occurrence of significant complications" related to PN and/or CIF.[63] A reasonable approach could argue for establishment of different thresholds for consideration of ITX, depending on the underlying cause for CIF and the potential for intestinal rehabilitation based on diagnosis

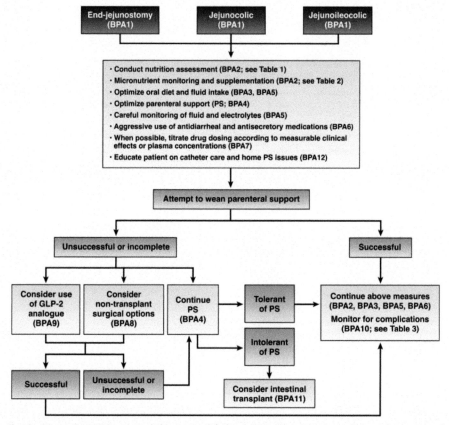

Fig. 2. Managing SBS-associated intestinal failure. BPA: Best Practice Advice; PS: Parenteral Support (*Reproduced* with permission from Iyer K, DiBaise JK, Rubio-Tapia A. AGA Clinical Practice Update on Management of Short Bowel Syndrome: Expert Review. Clin Gastroenterol Hepatol. 2022 Oct;20(10):2185 -2194.e2. https://doi.org/10.1016/j.cgh.2022.05.032. Epub 2022 Jun 11. PMID: 35700884.)

and, in the case of SBS, residual gastrointestinal anatomy. Thus, the patient with global gastrointestinal dysmotility from pseudo-obstruction with a poor QOL on HPN who is unable to eat or drink and requires ongoing gastrointestinal decompression through ostomies or enteric tubes could be considered early for ITX even before the onset of complications. Similarly, the patient with extreme SBS who has a stapled off foregut and requires foregut decompression through a gastrostomy tube while on PN has no potential for PN weaning and should rightfully be considered early for ITX, even pre-emptively. A proposed schema for a rational, multi-modality approach to the care of CIF with timely consideration of ITX is shown in (**Fig. 2**).

Ultimately, an enlightened approach may view ITX as perhaps the extreme tool in the ever-enlarging box of intestinal rehabilitation, and one that is best deployed in timely manner in a patient who can still expect good long-term survival with a good QOL.

CLINICS CARE POINTS

- Traditionally, intestinal transplant is reserved for patients with irreversible intestinal failure and complications of parenteral nutrition.
- The need for simultaneous liver replacement at the time of intestinal transplant, in most cases suggests late referral for transplant.
- Mortality on the waiting list is greater for patients awaiting combined liver and intestinal transplant, compared to patients awaiting isolated intestinal transplant.
- Early referral of patients with intestinal failure at high risk for parenteral nutrition-related complications or with poor quality fo life on parenteral nutrition may improve intestinal transplant outcomes.

DISCLOSURE

K.R. Iyer is a Scientific advisor and Consultant at Ironwood Pharmaceuticals and a Scientific advisor at Northsea Therapeutics and Hanmi Pharmaceuticals. K.R. Iyer received Grant support from Ironwood Pharmaceuticals, Takeda Pharmaceuticals, Northsea Therapeutics, and Hanmi Pharmaceuticals.

REFERENCES

1. Dudrick SJ, Wilmore DW, Vars HM, et al. Can intravenous feeding as the sole means of nutrition support growth in the child and restore weight loss in an adult? An affirmative answer. Ann Surg 1969;169(6):974–84.
2. Wilmore DW, Dudrick SJ. Safe long-term venous catheterization. Arch Surg 1969; 98(2):256–8.
3. Dudrick SJ, Wilmore DW, Vars HM, et al. Long-term total parenteral nutrition with growth, development, and positive nitrogen balance. Surgery 1968;64(1):134–42.
4. Pironi L, Arends J, Baxter J, et al. Home Artificial Nutrition & Chronic Intestinal Failure; Acute Intestinal Failure Special Interest Groups of ESPEN. ESPEN endorsed recommendations. Definition and classification of intestinal failure in adults. Clin Nutr 2015;34(2):171–80.
5. Howard L, Heaphey LL, Timchalk M. A review of the current national status of home parenteral and enteral nutrition from the provider and consumer perspective. JPEN J Parenter Enteral Nutr 1986;10(4):416–24.

6. Howard L. Home nutritional support: the patient point of view. Nutr Clin Pract 1989;4(2):49–50.
7. Baxter JP, Fayers PM, Bozzetti F, et al. Home Artificial Nutrition and Chronic Intestinal Failure Special Interest Group of the European Society for Clinical Nutrition and Metabolism (ESPEN). An international study of the quality of life of adult patients treated with home parenteral nutrition. Clin Nutr 2019;38(4):1788–96.
8. Winkler MF, Machan JT, Xue Z, et al. Home parenteral nutrition patient-reported outcome questionnaire: sensitive to quality of life differences among chronic and prolonged acute intestinal failure patients. JPEN J Parenter Enteral Nutr 2021;45(7):1475–83.
9. Winkler MF, Smith CE. The impact of long-term home parenteral nutrition on the patient and the family: achieving normalcy in life. J Infus Nurs 2015;38(4): 290–300.
10. Kelly DG, Tappenden KA, Winkler MF. Short bowel syndrome: highlights of patient management, quality of life, and survival. JPEN J Parenter Enteral Nutr 2014; 38(4):427–37.
11. Santarpia L, Buonomo A, Pagano MC, et al. Central venous catheter related bloodstream infections in adult patients on home parenteral nutrition: Prevalence, predictive factors, therapeutic outcome. Clin Nutr 2016;35(6):1394–8.
12. Pironi L, Corcos O, Forbes A, et al. ESPEN Acute and chronic intestinal failure special interest groups. intestinal failure in adults: recommendations from the ESPEN expert groups. Clin Nutr 2018;37(6 Pt A):1798–809.
13. Allan P, Stevens P, Chadwick P, et al. Osteomyelitis in adult patients on long-term parenteral nutrition: 2745 patient-years of experience in a national referral centre. Clin Nutr 2016;35(5):1135–9.
14. Huard G, Fiel MI, Moon J, et al. Prevalence, evolution, and risk factors for advanced liver fibrosis in adults undergoing intestinal transplantation. JPEN J Parenter Enteral Nutr 2018;42(7):1195–202.
15. Buchman AL, Iyer K, Fryer J. Parenteral nutrition-associated liver disease and the role for isolated intestine and intestine/liver transplantation. Hepatology 2006; 43(1):9–19.
16. Horslen SP, Sudan DL, Iyer KR, et al. Isolated liver transplantation in infants with end-stage liver disease associated with short bowel syndrome. Ann Surg 2002; 235(3):435–9.
17. Sasdelli AS, Agostini F, Pazzeschi C, et al. Assessment of intestinal failure associated liver disease according to different diagnostic criteria. Clin Nutr 2019; 38(3):1198–205.
18. Pironi L, Sasdelli AS. Intestinal failure-associated liver disease. Clin Liver Dis 2019;23(2):279–91.
19. Siddiqui MT, Al-Yaman W, Singh A, et al. Short-bowel syndrome: epidemiology, hospitalization trends, in-hospital mortality, and healthcare utilization. JPEN J Parenter Enteral Nutr 2021;45(7):1441–55.
20. Cavicchi M, Beau P, Crenn P, et al. Prevalence of liver disease and contributing factors in patients receiving home parenteral nutrition for permanent intestinal failure. Ann Intern Med 2000;132(7):525–32.
21. Joly F, Baxter J, Staun M, et al, ESPEN HAN CIF group. Five-year survival and causes of death in patients on home parenteral nutrition for severe chronic and benign intestinal failure. Clin Nutr 2018;37(4):1415–22.
22. Iyer KR, Kunecki M, Boullata JI, et al. Independence from parenteral nutrition and intravenous fluid support during treatment with teduglutide among patients with

intestinal failure associated with short bowel syndrome. JPEN J Parenter Enteral Nutr 2017;41(6):946–51.

23. Pape UF, Iyer KR, Jeppesen PB, et al. Teduglutide for the treatment of adults with intestinal failure associated with short bowel syndrome: pooled safety data from four clinical trials. Therap Adv Gastroenterol 2020;13. 1756284820905766.

24. Jeppesen PB, Pertkiewicz M, Messing B, et al. Teduglutide reduces need for parenteral support among patients with short bowel syndrome with intestinal failure. Gastroenterology 2012;143(6):1473–81, e3.

25. Grant D, Abu-Elmagd K, Mazariegos G, et al, Intestinal Transplant Association. Intestinal transplant registry report: global activity and trends. Am J Transplant 2015;15(1):210–9.

26. https://www.cms.gov/medicare/provider-enrollment-and-certification/guidancefor lawsandregulations/downloads/transplantfinallawandreg.pdf. [Accessed 18 February 2024].

27. https://www.cms.gov/medicare-coverage-database/view/ncd.aspx?ncdid=280. [Accessed 18 February 2024].

28. Howard L. Home parenteral nutrition: survival, cost, and quality of life. Gastroenterology 2006;130(2 Suppl 1):S52–9.

29. Howard L, Heaphey L, Fleming CR, et al. Four years of North American registry home parenteral nutrition outcome data and their implications for patient management. JPEN J Parenter Enteral Nutr 1991;15(4):384–93.

30. Ivanics T, Vianna R, Kubal CA, et al. Impact of the acuity circle model for liver allocation on multivisceral transplant candidates. Am J Transplant 2022;22(2):464–73.

31. Horslen SP, Smith JM, Weaver T, et al. OPTN/SRTR 2020 annual data report: intestine. Am J Transplant 2022;22(Suppl 2):310–49.

32. Rege A, Sudan D. Intestinal transplantation. Best Pract Res Clin Gastroenterol 2016;30(2):319–35.

33. Iyer K, Moon J. Adult intestinal transplantation in the United States. Curr Opin Organ Transplant 2020;25(2):196–200.

34. Hawksworth JS, Desai CS, Khan KM, et al. Visceral transplantation in patients with intestinal-failure associated liver disease: Evolving indications, graft selection, and outcomes. Am J Transplant 2018;18(6):1312–20.

35. Matsumoto CS, Subramanian S, Fishbein TM. Adult intestinal transplantation. Gastroenterol Clin North Am 2018;47(2):341–54.

36. Canovai E, Butler A, Clark S, et al. Treatment of complex desmoid tumors in familial adenomatous polyposis syndrome by intestinal transplantation. Transplant Direct 2024;10(2):e1571.

37. Chatzipetrou MA, Tzakis AG, Pinna AD, et al. Intestinal transplantation for the treatment of desmoid tumors associated with familial adenomatous polyposis. Surgery 2001;129(3):277–81.

38. Wheeler M, Mercer D, Grant W, et al. Surgical treatment of intra-abdominal desmoid tumors resulting in short bowel syndrome. Cancers (Basel) 2012;4(1):31–8.

39. Moon JI, Selvaggi G, Nishida S, et al. Intestinal transplantation for the treatment of neoplastic disease. J Surg Oncol 2005;92(4):284–91.

40. Pironi L, Hébuterne X, Van Gossum A, et al. Candidates for intestinal transplantation: a multicenter survey in Europe. Am J Gastroenterol 2006;101(7):1633–43, quiz 1679.

41. Pironi L, Forbes A, Joly F, et al. Home artificial nutrition working group of the european society for clinical nutrition and metabolism (ESPEN). survival of patients

identified as candidates for intestinal transplantation: a 3-year prospective follow-up. Gastroenterology 2008;135(1):61–71.

42. Pironi L, Joly F, Forbes A, et al. Home artificial nutrition & chronic intestinal failure working group of the european society for clinical nutrition and metabolism (ESPEN). Long-term follow-up of patients on home parenteral nutrition in Europe: implications for intestinal transplantation. Gut 2011;60(1):17–25.

43. Kaufman SS, Avitzur Y, Beath SV, et al. New insights into the indications for intestinal transplantation: consensus in the year 2019. Transplantation 2020;104(5): 937–46.

44. Horslen SP, Smith JM, Ahn Y, et al. OPTN/SRTR 2019 annual data report: intestine. Am J Transplant 2021 Feb;21(Suppl 2):316–55.

45. Smith JM, Weaver T, Skeans MA, et al. OPTN/SRTR 2016 annual data report: intestine. Am J Transplant 2018;18(Suppl 1):254–90.

46. Pironi L, Sasdelli AS. New insights into the indications for intestinal transplantation. Curr Opin Organ Transplant 2021;26(2):186–91.

47. Mangus RS, Tector AJ, Kubal CA, et al. Multivisceral transplantation: expanding indications and improving outcomes. J Gastrointest Surg 2013;17(1):179–86, discussion p.186-7.

48. Vianna RM, Mangus RS, Kubal C, et al. Multivisceral transplantation for diffuse portomesenteric thrombosis. Ann Surg 2012 Jun;255(6):1144–50.

49. Kaufman SS, Atkinson JB, Bianchi A, et al. Indications for pediatric intestinal transplantation: a position paper of the American Society of Transplantation. Pediatr Transplant 2001;5(2):80–7.

50. Burghardt KM, Wales PW, de Silva N, et al. Pediatric intestinal transplant listing criteria - a call for a change in the new era of intestinal failure outcomes. Am J Transplant 2015;15(6):1674–81.

51. Roberts AJ, Wales PW, Beath SV, et al. An international multicenter validation study of the Toronto listing criteria for pediatric intestinal transplantation. Am J Transplant 2022;22(11):2608–15.

52. Huard G, Schiano TD, Moon J, et al. Severe acute cellular rejection after intestinal transplantation is associated with poor patient and graft survival. Clin Transplant 2017;31(5). https://doi.org/10.1111/ctr.12956.

53. Ganoza A, Celik N, Mazariegos GV. Intestinal re-transplantation: indications, techniques and outcomes. Curr Opin Organ Transplant 2018;23(2):224–8.

54. Ekser B, Kubal CA, Fridell JA, et al. Comparable outcomes in intestinal retransplantation: Single-center cohort study. Clin Transplant 2018;32(7):e13290.

55. Iyer KR, Horslen S, Torres C, et al. Functional liver recovery parallels autologous gut salvage in short bowel syndrome. J Pediatr Surg 2004;39(3):340–4, discussion 340-4.

56. Nucci A, Burns RC, Armah T, et al. Interdisciplinary management of pediatric intestinal failure: a 10-year review of rehabilitation and transplantation. J Gastrointest Surg 2008;12(3):429–35, discussion 435-6.

57. Iyer K, DiBaise JK, Rubio-Tapia A. AGA clinical practice update on management of short bowel syndrome: expert review. Clin Gastroenterol Hepatol 2022;20(10): 2185–94.e2.

58. Messing B, Crenn P, Beau P, et al. Long-term survival and parenteral nutrition dependence in adult patients with the short bowel syndrome. Gastroenterology 1999;117(5):1043–50.

59. Amiot A, Messing B, Corcos O, et al. Determinants of home parenteral nutrition dependence and survival of 268 patients with non-malignant short bowel syndrome. Clin Nutr 2013;32(3):368–74.

60. Pironi L, Steiger E, Joly F, et al. Intravenous supplementation type and volume are associated with 1-year outcome and major complications in patients with chronic intestinal failure. Gut 2020;69(10):1787–95.
61. Fullerton BS, Sparks EA, Hall AM, et al. Enteral autonomy, cirrhosis, and long term transplant-free survival in pediatric intestinal failure patients. J Pediatr Surg 2016; 51(1):96–100.
62. Khan FA, Squires RH, Litman HJ, et al. Pediatric intestinal failure consortium. predictors of enteral autonomy in children with intestinal failure: a multicenter cohort study. J Pediatr 2015;167(1):29–34.e1.
63. Lauro A, Marino IR, Iyer KR. Pre-emptive intestinal transplant: the surgeon's point of view. Dig Dis Sci 2017;62(11):2966–76.

Indications for Multivisceral Transplantation
A Systematic Review

Pierpaolo Di Cocco, MD, PhD[a], Alessandro Martinino, MD[a,*],
Amy Lian, BS[b], Jess Johnson, BS[b], Mario Spaggiari, MD[a],
Ivo Tzvetanov, MD[a], Enrico Benedetti, MD[a]

KEYWORDS

- Indications • Intestinal failure • Multivisceral transplantation

KEY POINTS

- A systematic review with the goal of gathering and synthesizing the available literature on indications for multivisceral transplantation (MVT).
- Consensus remains elusive in the definition and indications of MVT within the transplant community.
- The management of this patient population remains challenging with a fine balance between immunosuppression and infection

INTRODUCTION

Multivisceral transplant (MVT) as a concept was first introduced by Thomas Starzl in the 1960s, originally performed on dogs.[1] The first 2 human cases were performed in the 1980s; however, the outcomes were dismal; one patient died perioperatively and the other patient died 6-months post-transplant from an Epstein-Barr virus (EBV)–associated lymphoproliferative disorder.[2]

There is not yet consensus regarding the exact definition of MVT as a subset of intestinal transplantation. In MVT, many different organ combinations are possible and it is usually referred to as transplantation of all organs dependent on the celiac artery axis and the superior mesenteric artery (SMA), which includes the stomach, liver, pancreas, duodenum, and jejunoileum. Several classifications are present in the literature; the most widely used for its simplicity is the one that categorizes MVT as "classical" or "full" if it includes the liver or "modified" MVT (MMVT) if the liver is excluded.[3]

[a] Division of Transplantation, Department of Surgery, University of Illinois at Chicago, Chicago, IL, USA; [b] University of Illinois at Chicago College of Medicine, Chicago, IL, USA
* Corresponding author. Department of Surgery, University of Illinois at Chicago, 840 South Wood Street, Suite 502, Clinical Science Building, Chicago, IL, 60612.
E-mail address: alessandro.martinino@gmail.com

Advances in immunosuppression and medical management have been a crucial contributor to the expansion and improved outcomes of MVT. However, the management of this patient population remains challenging with a fine balance between immunosuppression and infection and an increased incidence of graft-versus-host-disease (GVHD) and posttransplant lymphoproliferative disorder (PTLD) compared to other solid-organ transplants.[4,5]

MVT indications include the broad categories of intestinal failure, tumors, intestinal dysmotility disorders, and trauma. Intestinal failure is the inability of the native bowel to adequately absorb fluid, electrolytes, and major nutrients due to decreased absorptive surface and/or impaired function of the small bowel.[4] The most common cause of intestinal failure is short gut syndrome, which results from loss of most of the small intestine. Consideration is given to MVT when specific organs, besides the small bowel, have underlying pathology nonresponsive to medical therapy or nonresectable with traditional surgical procedures.[6]

The aim of this systematic review is to summarize the existing literature describing the indications for MVT.

METHODS

In the context of this investigation, the authors undertook a comprehensive and systematic literature search to identify articles discussing the indications for MVT. The authors conducted a thorough analysis of the current clinical landscape, augmented by an expert review, with the goal of offering a comprehensive assessment of the contemporary medical imperatives driving MVTs. This holistic approach aimed to enhance understanding of the subject and contribute valuable insights to the medical community.

Search Strategy

Our research encompassed an exhaustive computerized exploration of the PubMed and Cochrane Library databases. The following search terms were used "multivisceral transplantation," "multiorgan transplantation," "complex organ transplantation," and "combined transplantation." Articles were also identified from references of the published articles. The last of these searches were carried out on the seventh of May 2023.

Inclusion and Exclusion Criteria

All published English language studies, including cohort studies, case series, case reports, and reviews, were included. The authors excluded all non-English language studies. Moreover, articles discussing single-organ transplantation were excluded. This stringent approach ensured that our analysis was focused solely on sources that provided relevant insights and information pertaining to the topic at hand, enhancing the precision and relevance of our research findings.

Study Selection

Titles and/or abstracts of studies identified using our search criteria were screened independently by 2 authors (AM & AL) to identify all studies meeting our inclusion criteria. Any disagreement was resolved through discussion with a third reviewer (GB). A total of 144 studies were assessed for eligibility by reviewing the full text. **Fig. 1** provides the Preferred Reporting Items for Systematic Reviews and Meta-Analyses (PRISMA) flow chart for this. The authors did not perform a meta-analysis because of inconsistent reporting of outcome measures and differences in populations and study design.

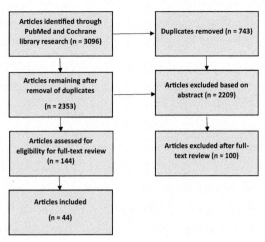

Fig. 1. Preferred Reporting Items for Systematic Reviews and Meta-Analyses (PRISMA) flow diagram.

Data Extraction

Two authors (AL & GB) reviewed the full texts for inclusion and data extraction. AM then reviewed all 44 articles, rechecked data, and analyzed them using an Excel(R) sheet. A total of 44 studies were deemed eligible for inclusion (**Table 1**).

RESULTS
Results of the Search Strategy

Our initial search resulted in 3096 articles. After removing duplicates, title and abstract screening, and full-text assessment as needed, 2353 articles published by May 2023 were identified for inclusion in this review. A total of 44 articles were included. **Fig. 1** highlights our search strategy and the PRISMA flow diagram. In terms of study design, a total of 15 were case series, 8 were retrospective cohort studies, and 21 were case reports. The study characteristics are shown in **Table 1**. The findings are succinctly outlined and organized chronologically within each subgroup (whenever applicable), in accordance with the indications for MVT.

Indication for Multivisceral Transplant: Tumor

MVT or MMVT has been reported in the treatment of patients with nonresectable slow-growing tumors involving the mesenteric root, with local recurrence after failure of conventional medical or surgical therapy, and with intestinal failure due to short bowel syndrome (SBS) secondary to previous tumor resections. First described in 1989 by Starzl and colleagues,[7] it appears to be a good and, sometimes, the only therapeutic option for this group of patients. Given the rarity of these conditions and the even rarer number of transplant centers performing MVT and MMVT, data from the literature present the limitations of single-center and retrospective analyses.[8]

In a retrospective study of 100 MVTs between 2004 and 2010 at Indiana University, 11 cases had a surgical indication of nonresectable tumor including desmoid tumors, metastatic neuroendocrine tumors (NETs), schwannoma, and hepatoblastoma.[6] These patients all had either involvement of mesenteric root vasculature or metastases to the liver, without peritoneal or extra-abdominal involvement. Two patients with gastrointestinal stromal tumors (GISTs) successfully underwent MMVT. All

Table 1
Study characteristics

Author, Year	Type of Study	Indication for Multivisceral Transplantation
Masetti et al,[40] 1999	Case series	Dysmotility (n = 3) [a]
Vennarecci et al,[48] 2000	Case series	Pediatric condition (n = 3)
Kornberg et al,[21] 2001	Case series	Tumor (n = 3)
Olausson et al,[26] 2001	Case report	Ischemia (n = 1)
Florman et al,[25] 2002	Case report	Ischemia (n = 1)
Jovine et al,[13] 2002	Retrospective cohort	Dysmotility (n = 1), tumor (n = 1)
Olausson et al,[20] 2002	Case series	Tumor (n = 2)
Loinaz et al,[33] 2004	Case series	Dysmotility (n = 16) [a]
Nishida et al,[32] 2004	Case series	Trauma (n = 5) [b]
Loinaz et al,[34] 2005	Case series	Dysmotility (n = 11) [a]
López-Santamaría et al,[35] 2005	Case report	Dysmotility (n = 1)
Tryphonopoulos et al,[10] 2005	Case series	Tumor (n = 3) [c]
Tzakis et al,[5] 2005	Retrospective cohort	Dysmotility (n = 24) [a], ischemia (n = 14), pediatric condition (n = 42), trauma (n = 5) [b], tumor (n = 5) [c], other (n = 8)
Vianna et al,[27] 2005	Case report	Ischemia (n = 1)
Pascher et al,[52] 2006	Case report	Other (n = 1)
Takahashi et al,[36] 2006	Case report	Dysmotility (n = 1)
Nathan et al,[41] 2007	Retrospective cohort	Pediatric condition (n = 4), dysmotility (n = 1)
Takahashi et al,[46] 2007	Case report	Dysmotility (n = 1)
Koh et al,[37] 2008	Case report	Dysmotility (n = 1)
Cruz et al,[12] 2010	Retrospective cohort	Dysmotility (n = 19), tumor (n = 6), ischemia (n = 1), other (n = 10)
Bauschke et al,[53] 2012	Case report	Tumor (n = 1)
Cauley et al,[49] 2012	Case report	Pediatric condition (n = 1)
Ravindra et al,[42] 2012	Case report	Dysmotility (n = 1), pediatric condition (n = 1)
Vianna et al,[24] 2012	Case series	Ischemia (n = 25)
Lauro et al,[38] 2013	Case series	Dysmotility (n = 2)
Mangus et al,[6,d] 2013	Retrospective cohort	Tumor (n = 11), ischemia (n = 34), dysmotility (n = 7), other (n = 48)
Nikeghbalian et al,[15] 2014	Retrospective cohort	Ischemia (n = 2), tumor (n = 9), trauma (n = 1), other (n = 2)
Vakili et al,[17] 2014	Case report	Tumor (n = 1)
Girlanda et al,[51] 2016	Case report	Other (n = 1)
Koval et al,[28] 2016	Case report	Ischemia (n = 1)
Moulin et al,[19] 2016	Case report	Tumor (n = 1)
Moulin et al,[22] 2016	Case report	Tumor (n = 1)
Samuk et al,[14] 2016	Retrospective cohort	Tumor (n = 2), other (n = 1)

(continued on next page)

Table 1
(continued)

Author, Year	Type of Study	Indication for Multivisceral Transplantation
Sharkey et al,[31] 2016	Case series	Ischemia (n = 3)
Clift et al,[18] 2017	Case report	Tumor (n = 1)
Chi et al,[9,d] 2018	Case series	Tumor (n = 6)
Janousek et al,[11] 2019	Case report	Tumor (n = 1)
Nicolau-Raducu et al,[29] 2019	Case series	Ischemia (n = 3)
Kunzler de Oliveira Maia et al,[43] 2020	Retrospective cohort	Pediatric condition (n = 1), dysmotility (n = 1), other (n = 1)
Canovai et al,[23] 2021	Case series	Ischemia (n = 5)
Estefanía-Fernández K et al,[50] 2022	Case report	Pediatric condition (n = 1)
Grosman et al,[39] 2022	Case report	Dysmotility (n = 1)
Livingstone et al,[30] 2022	Case report	Ischemia (n = 1)
Reddy et al,[16] 2022	Case series	Tumor (n = 7)

[a] The 3 patients in the Masetti and colleagues' 1999 study are included in the Loinaz and colleagues' 2004 study as well. There is also an unclear redundancy between the patients in Loinaz and colleagues' 2004 study and Loinaz and colleagues' 2005 study. The patients from these studies are all from the University of Miami, of which the study by Tzakis and colleagues (2005) is a comprehensive review.
[b] The 5 trauma patients in these 2 studies appear to be the same patients, as they are from the same center during the same period.
[c] Tryphonopoulos and colleagues (2005) describe 3 of the tumor cases in Tzakis and colleagues' 2005 study in greater detail.
[d] There is unclear overlap between these 2 studies, as they are from the same center with partially overlapping time periods.

patients with NETs had diffuse liver involvement. The authors reported a recurrence rate of 27% (3 of 11 patients): 1 sarcoma (recurrence at 10 months, survived 16 months), 1 carcinoid (recurrence at 10 months, survived 10 months), and 1 gastrinoma (recurrence at 23 months, alive at 40 months) with an overall patient survival rate of 82%.

Intra-abdominal fibromatosis as an indication for MVT is better described in a study by Chi and colleagues[9] that reviewed 6 patients at Indiana University between 2005 and 2015. Intra-abdominal fibromatosis (desmoid tumor) is locally aggressive and often involves the bowel or mesentery root. A wide resection with a negative surgical margin cannot always be achieved; there is a high rate of recurrence, and SBS can result due to repeated surgeries. Patients often need total parenteral nutrition (TPN), and ultimately transplantation is indicated for patients with nonresectable tumors or who develop complications of TPN.[10] The 6 patients in this study, of whom 4 had familial adenomatous polyposis, all had a primary tumor site in the mesentery. In this contest, autologous reconstruction of SMA base, autotransplantation, or ex vivo resection were not options, leaving MVT as the last-line option for what would otherwise be a fatal condition.[9]

Janousek and colleagues[11] report on a patient with Gardner's syndrome with a history of abdominal surgery who was diagnosed with mesenteric fibromatosis that embedded the uterus, internal and external iliac vessels, and celiac and mesenteric arteries. She had normal kidney function and nonalcoholic steatohepatitis. MVT with kidney autotransplantation was chosen for this patient including a liver graft due to the progressive nature of liver fibrosis and the patient's previous history of multiple abdominal surgeries. She had no graft rejection or evidence of disease recurrence after a 1-year follow-up.[11] While this patient had classical MVT including the liver, a different study at the University of Pittsburgh includes 6 patients with Gardner's syndrome who received MMVT for extensive desmoid tumors involving the main mesenteric vascular pedicle, pancreas, and duodenum with failed previous attempts of resection or autotransplantation. Similarly, a patient with Gardner's syndrome and normal liver function underwent MMVT at the University of Modena in Italy due to diffuse gastric involvement and presence of desmoid lesions at the mesenteric root and around the pancreas. Indeed, Cruz and colleagues[12] and Jovine and colleagues[13] state that with preserved hepatic function and in the absence of portal hypertension, MMVT can be safely offered to patients with diffuse gastrointestinal (GI) disorders primarily involving the hollow viscera including the stomach, duodenum, and intestine, including Gardner's syndrome.

Tryphonopoulos and colleagues[10] describe 3 patients who had MVT for intra-abdominal fibromatosis at the University of Miami. Patient 1 received MVT but died within 1 month due to unspecified postoperative complications. Patient 2 received MVT with kidney and patient 3 received MMVT with abdominal wall graft due to desmoid tumors involving the recipient abdominal wall. They had transitioned to enteral nutrition and were alive at 9-year and 1-year follow-up, respectively. These 3 patients are also included in the study by Tzakis and colleagues[5] reporting on 98 patients who underwent primary MVT between December 1994 and April 2005 at the University of Miami.

Another study reported on pediatric patients at the University of Miami who underwent abdominal transplantation for a neoplasm between June 1994 and September 2010, with 2 patients receiving MVT. A 32-month-old male had hepatoblastoma status post (s/p) right hepatectomy at age 1 that recurred 16 months later with portal vein (PV) involvement. He received MVT because it offered better oncological margins than liver transplant alone due to PV involvement and addressed SBS. He was alive at the 52-month follow-up. The second patient was an 8.5-year-old female with pancreatic blastoma, PV tumor thrombosis, and liver metastases, with the indication for MVT being PV tumor invasion. She died of lung metastases 12 months post-transplantation[14]

In a retrospective study at Shiraz Organ Transplant Center in Iran, 6 patients had MVT for desmoid tumor (n = 1), hepatocellular carcinoma (HCC) (n = 1), NET (n = 2), pancreatic carcinoma (n = 1), and small round cell tumor (n = 1). MMVT was performed for GIST (n = 2) and pancreatic carcinoma (n = 1). For the patients with HCC or pancreatic carcinoma, MVT or MMVT was performed due to tumors being locally advanced and unresectable due to anatomic limitations such as SMA involvement. The patient with HCC underwent MVT due to hilar involvement.[15]

A study at Oxford by Reddy and colleagues[16] describes intestinal transplant or MMVT in 15 patients with pseudomyxoma peritonei (PMP) and nutrition failure, not amenable to further surgery, of which 7 patients received MMVT of the stomach, pancreaticoduodenal complex, small bowel, and right colon. The reported patient selection criteria included young age, low-grade disease, fit enough to undergo extensive surgery, and ensuring no possible conventional operative approaches. In this cohort, 2 patients died within 3 months after surgery, 2 patients had PMP recurrence, and 1 patient had graft failure requiring restarting TPN.[16]

An interesting case report by Vakili and colleagues[17] discusses a pediatric patient with an inflammatory myofibroblastic tumor involving the upper retroperitoneum, visceral vessels, stomach, and distal esophagus, who received MVT at age 9 at Boston Children's Hospital after failed initial resection. At the time of initial resection, she had celiac trunk (CT) involvement, which prevented complete resection and led to tumor progression. She underwent a gastrojejunostomy but continued to have slow tumor progression with failed maximal medical therapy, leading to ascites, recurrent upper GI bleeding, and feeding difficulties by age 8. MVT at age 9 interestingly included resection of the distal third of recipient esophagus due to tumor involvement. At 1.9 years, surveillance computed tomography scans demonstrated no evidence of tumor recurrence, and the patient was tolerating oral intake without dysphagia or reflux symptoms.[17]

A case report by Clift and colleagues[18] discusses a 44-year-old male, with well-differentiated NET within the small bowel mesentery and extensive lymph node metastases that was not amenable to conventional surgical approaches, who received MMVT at Oxford Transplant Center, Oxford, UK. At the time of the procedure, the mass in the root of the mesentery involved the duodenum and pancreas and a lymph node in the aortocaval groove but not the liver. At 48 months post-transplantation, he was on full enteral nutrition.

A case report by Moulin and colleagues[19] describes a 7-year-old female with mesenteric root localization of cystic lymphangioma, causing intestinal failure due to venous congestion. The tumor was unresponsive to chemotherapy, and the tumor was nonresectable due to multivisceral involvement and involvement of the mesenteric root. She had a fully functioning graft at discharge on postoperative day (POD) 36. However, she was readmitted 3 months post-transplant with a severe EBV infection leading to severe PTLD with central nervous system effects, from which she eventually died.

Two patients in a study by Olausson and colleagues[20] received MVT for endocrine pancreatic tumors at the head of the pancreas with lymph node and liver involvement; both patients had large tumor burdens (>50%). One patient was diagnosed with recurrent disease 15 months post-transplant; however, he was asymptomatic, and further surgery was not planned. The second patient died 4 months post-transplant from PTLD induced by immunosuppression, but no evidence of tumor recurrence was found on autopsy.

Three patients in another study by Kornberg and colleagues[21] received MVT for malignant abdominal tumors. Patient 1 had multiple peritoneal and mesenterial metastases of a recurrent malignant GIST of the ileum s/p 2 resections. MVT was performed to best guarantee complete tumor removal. Nineteen months postoperatively, this patient required removal of a soft-tissue metastasis in the right groin. Later, the patient required pancreas-kidney transplantation due to Tac-induced nephropathy and diabetes mellitus due to pancreas graft dysfunction. At the last follow-up, the patient was free of tumors and on complete enteral nutrition. This case is the first reported metastatic malignant GIST of the ileum successfully treated with MVT. Patient 2 had recurrent NET of the bile duct; after the transplant she was free of tumor and on total enteral nutrition. Patient 3 had nonresectable aggressive desmoid fibromatosis infiltrating mesenterial and celiac vascular structures s/p gastrectomy, partial pancreatectomy, and colectomy due to low-grade sarcoma of the stomach. The patient died 9 months after MVT due to severe EBV and herpes simplex virus infection. Kornberg and colleagues[12] state MVT may be a last-line curative option for nonresectable malignant abdominal tumors in select compliant patients. Similarly, Moulin and colleagues[22] state the presence of high-grade dysplasia should be considered the primary indication for transplantation as the only curative option, even in the absence of intestinal failure. They present a patient with Peutz-Jeghers syndrome with greater than 150 polyps, some with high-grade dysplasia, at the time of MMVT. He had previously undergone 8 surgeries but maintained intestinal sufficiency and he was listed for MMVT to avoid future complications of Peutz-Jeghers syndrome and cancer development. He was alive at the 23-month follow-up.

Indication for Multivisceral Transplant: Ischemia

Portomesenteric thrombosis

Diffuse portomesenteric thrombosis (PMT), defined as the complete occlusion of the portal system, is one of the most common indications for MVT.[23] For patients with diffuse PMT, liver transplant alone may fail to reverse the patient's portal hypertension. MVT is a viable treatment option for these patients by replacing the entire portomesenteric venous system, allowing for reversal of portal hypertension and its sequelae.[24]

Florman and colleagues[25] report a case of MVT performed for diffuse visceral splanchnic thrombosis secondary to protein C deficiency. Mesenteric thrombosis is not a common sequela of protein C deficiency, though it usually occurs late in the disease process if it does occur. The patient was a 25-year-old previously healthy male who presented with acute abdominal pain and underwent exploratory laparotomy. During surgery, a segment of the small intestine was found to be thrombosed and was excised. He presented 9 years later with acute GI hemorrhage and was found to have large duodenal varices. Imaging revealed prehepatic mesenteric thrombosis. Embolization of the splenic artery ultimately failed to control the bleeding, and transjugular intrahepatic portosystemic shunt placement was prevented by extensive PMT. Hypercoagulability workup was significant for severe protein C deficiency and the patient was begun on anticoagulation. The patient was listed for MVT after he continued to have episodes of life-threatening variceal bleeding. The graft consisted of the stomach, pancreas, liver, and small bowel. The patient's protein C level increased from undetectable prior to transplant to 55 U/dL on POD 2 and greater than 100 U/dL on POD 14 (normal level: 70–140 U/dL). He was discharged home 6 weeks after transplantation and was doing well at the follow-up at 17 months.[25]

A case report from Göteborg (Sweden) describes the course of a female patient who underwent MVT at 5 years of age. She was referred for MVT after developing TPN-related hepatic complications, central vein thrombosis, and life-threatening septicemia. The donor graft consisted of the stomach, duodenum, liver, pancreas, and small bowel. Her postoperative course was complicated by acute rejection requiring resection of a 25-cm section of the distal ileum, as well as later intussusception requiring an additional surgery. She was doing well at the 18-month follow-up.[26]

In 2005, Vianna and colleagues[27] reported an individual case of a 26-year-old male undergoing MVT for refractory gastroesophageal variceal bleeding secondary to extrahepatic portal hypertension, in turn secondary to PMT. The en bloc graft included the stomach, liver, pancreas, and small bowel. Twelve months after transplantation, the patient had not experienced any major complications.[27] A retrospective analysis from the same center examined all 25 cases of MVT indicated for PMT from 2004 to 2009. One patient died within 30 days of transplantation, and 5 patients died within the first year, giving a 1-year survival rate of 80%. The survival rate was 72% at 3 and 5 years.[24]

Between 2004 and 2010, 34 patients underwent MVT for PMT at Indiana University. Thirty-three of these were adults. If indicated, several of the operations included a simultaneous kidney transplant.[6]

In a retrospective analysis of MVT cases from 2010 to 2012 at Shiraz University in Iran, 1 patient underwent MVT for liver cirrhosis with extensive PMT and superior mesenteric vein (SMV) thrombosis and 1 patient underwent MMVT for SBS secondary to venous thrombosis.[15]

Koval and colleagues[28] published a case of a patient with human immunodeficiency virus (HIV) who underwent MVT for diffuse PMT. The patient initially presented with *Clostridium difficile* colitis, was found to be HIV-1 positive, and underwent a total colectomy with midgut resection for mesenteric venous infarction. He was placed on TPN and subsequently developed PMT a year later. The patient was placed on highly active antiretroviral therapy ahead of transplantation. The en bloc donor graft consisted of the stomach, duodenum, pancreas, intestine, and liver, as well as the right kidney. The patient died of systemic sepsis 2 months post-transplantation.[28]

Twenty-seven MVTs were performed at the University of Miami from 2014 to 2018. Twelve of these patients had stage IV PMT; of those, 3 underwent visceral arterial embolization prior to surgery due to being at exceptionally high risk of massive hemorrhage. Patient 1 had a history of liver transplant for hepatitis C and end-stage liver disease (ESLD) 14 years prior to presentation. He had recurrence of ESLD with PMT secondary to chronic rejection, hepatitis C, and chronic kidney disease. His embolization targeted the entire CT and SMA. He died intraoperatively of disseminated intravascular coagulation with extensive intracardiac thrombosis. Patient 2 had a long history of ulcerative colitis (UC) and primary sclerosing cholangitis (PSC), who underwent liver transplant with Roux-en-Y hepaticojejunostomy 9 years prior to presentation; he underwent a total proctocolectomy 6 years prior to presentation for a severe UC flare. He then developed ESLD with PMT secondary to PSC, which led to his presentation for MVT. His preoperative embolization targeted all end branches of the SMA distal to the origin of the inferior pancreaticoduodenal artery, the splenic artery, and the gastric artery. The recipient had a normal graft function at the 13-month follow-up. Patient 3 presented a history of cryptogenic cirrhosis and PMT. His prior surgical history included a small-bowel resection due to volvulus and incarcerated internal hernia 16 years prior to presentation. His embolization targeted all branches of the SMA and the gastroduodenal artery as well as the splenic artery. The patient recovered with no postoperative complications.[29]

In a retrospective analysis, Canovai and colleagues[23] report 5 cases of MVT performed for PMT from 2000 to 2020 at the University Hospitals in Leuven, Belgium. All 5 patients had diffuse PMT with recurrent life-threatening GI bleeding. In addition, patient 2 had intestinal failure and recurrent ascites. Patient 3 had severe liver disease and renal failure. One patient developed symptomatic grade III rejection that was refractory to treatment and underwent a partial graft enterectomy on POD 67. He died 254 days post-transplantation of cerebral hemorrhage secondary to rupture of a cerebral mycotic aneurysm from multifocal invasive aspergillosis. Four out of 5 patients survived with normal graft function at a mean follow-up of 4.1 years.[23]

A case report from Livingstone and colleagues[30] focuses on a female patient who underwent MVT at 29 years of age for PMT and porto-pulmonary hypertension (PPHTN). She received a liver transplant in infancy for biliary atresia. At 24 years of age, while taking oral contraception, she developed a deep vein thrombosis and progressive PMT that required 6 months of anticoagulation and then a splenorenal shunt followed by a mesocaval shunt both of which eventually thrombosed. An ensuing thrombophilic workup revealed abnormalities associated with cirrhosis. At 27 year old, she developed progressive shortness of breath and was diagnosed with PPHTN. The donor graft included the liver, stomach, pancreaticoduodenal complex, small intestine, and a segment of the colon. She was discharged to home 90 days after transplantation.[30]

Occlusion of celiac trunk and/or superior mesenteric artery

Sharkey and colleagues[31] describe 3 cases that offer support for complete occlusion of the SMA and/or CT as an indication for urgent MVT. Acute occlusion of the CT and concurrent occlusion of the SMA and CT have rarely been reported. Historically, if revascularization efforts failed, the only option available to patients with concurrent occlusion was palliative care. Patient 1 was a 33-year-old female that presented with acute occlusion of the CT, SMA, and inferior mesenteric artery. She had already undergone extensive small-bowel resection and attempted revascularization of the ileocolic and middle colic arteries without success; repeat laparotomy showed ischemia of the remaining small bowel and the ascending colon, along with areas of hepatic infarction. Completion enterectomy and right hemicolectomy were then performed, and she was given a venting gastrostomy. She was then referred for urgent MVT. Patient 2, a 48-year-old woman, presented with a small-bowel infarct secondary to SMA occlusion. She was placed on TPN and anticoagulation after undergoing enterotomy. Ten months later, she presented with acute liver failure with encephalopathy, coagulopathy, and sepsis. She was found to have occlusion of the CT on imaging and was listed for urgent MVT. Patient 3 was a 50-year-old woman who presented with occlusion of the SMA. After failing an attempt at revascularization via stent, she underwent extensive enterectomy and was placed on TPN. She presented 4 months later with ischemic liver abscesses and evidence of CT occlusion on imaging. She was subsequently listed for urgent MVT. The patients received grafts that included the stomach, liver, pancreas, small bowel, and colon. While patient 1 developed no acute postoperative complications, patient 2 had primary nonfunction of the liver graft that required retransplantation of the entire bloc on POD 2. Patient 3's postoperative course was complicated by GVHD with myelosuppression and resistant cytomegalovirus (CMV) infection. She died 8 months after transplantation.[31]

Indication for Multivisceral Transplant: Trauma

Severe trauma involving abdominal organs, particularly from mechanisms of injury such as motor vehicle crashes (MVCs) or gunshot wounds (GSWs), often requires emergency surgical interventions as lifesaving measures. SBS and other complications may result from the primary procedure(s), resulting in the need for MVT.

The Tzakis and colleagues'[5] study indicates 5 patients who received MVT for trauma, which are better described in another study by Nishida and colleagues.[32] This study was a retrospective review of 10 patients (8 adults and 2 pediatric patients) who received intestinal transplant and MVT after severe abdominal trauma at the University of Miami, of whom 5 patients underwent MVT. Patient 2 suffered SMA transection after an MVC. He initially underwent SMA revascularization, small-bowel resection, and right hemicolectomy, with the outcome of SBS, pancreatitis, liver failure, and open wound. Two years after MVT, he developed renal failure requiring a kidney transplant but was alive at the last follow-up on day 1327. Patient 3 suffered SMA and SMV injuries and pancreas crush injuries after an MVC. He developed SBS and open abdominal wound after initial surgeries including pancreaticoduodenectomy, splenectomy, gastric pouch, small-bowel resection, and right hemicolectomy. He was alive at the last follow-up on day 679 after MMVT. Both surviving patients are at home in good condition on a regular diet with good quality of life at the last follow-up. Patient 7 had vena cava and renal vein injuries and abdominal compartment syndrome after sustaining a GSW. He developed SBS, liver failure, renal failure, and an open wound after initially undergoing vena cava ligation, bilateral renal vein ligation, small-bowel resection, right hemicolectomy, and cholecystectomy. After MVT, he experienced moderate intestinal graft rejection in the first week, which was treated with OKT3 with good response. Antiviral and antifungal therapy was complicated by renal failure and thrombosis of all major veins, resulting in the need for a transhepatic catheter for hemodialysis. He died of CMV encephalitis 91 days after transplant. Patient 9 sustained SMA injuries after a GSW. He initially underwent small bowel resection and right hemicolectomy but developed SBS, pancreatitis, and liver failure. He had an episode of severe intestinal graft rejection during week 4, which was treated with OKT3. However, he developed translocation-associated severe sepsis, bilateral pneumonia, adenovirus infection, and renal failure. He died of sepsis 53 days post-transplant. Patient 10 sustained SMA and SMV injuries after MVC. He initially underwent small-bowel resection, right hemicolectomy, and cholecystectomy but developed SBS, liver failure, and portal hypertension. Of note, this patient was intensive care unit–bound before transplantation and was very unstable during surgery. He developed intestinal graft dysfunction, severe graft pancreatitis, and sepsis refractory to therapy and died on day 7 from pancreatitis and multiple organ failure (MOF).[32]

Nikeghbalian and colleagues[15] describe 1 patient who received MMVT for unspecified abdominal trauma; this patient was alive at the 17-month follow-up.

Indication for Multivisceral Transplant: Intestinal Dysmotility Syndromes

Chronic intestinal pseudo-obstruction

Chronic intestinal pseudo-obstruction (CIPO), characterized by symptoms of intestinal obstruction in the absence of mechanical obstruction, is a relatively rare condition for which transplant may be indicated if patients cannot safely begin or continue parental nutrition.[33] In the pediatric population, CIPO is usually primary; in adults, it is often secondary to various disorders such as muscular dystrophies and chronic infections.[34]

In a retrospective review from the University of Miami, Loinaz and colleagues[33,34] reported the cases of 8 pediatric patients who underwent MVT for CIPO between 1996 and 2004. The patients were parenteral nutrition (PN)–dependent and ultimately required surgery due to either liver disease, loss of venous access, or sepsis. The same center published a report the following year that included 4 cases of MVT indicated for CIPO between 1994 and 2001; there is likely overlap between these 2 papers.

At the University of Modena in Italy between 2000 and 2001, 1 patient with CIPO and normal liver function received an MVT. This patient was hospitalized for a total of 41 days and was able to gain normal intestinal function without TPN and with complete dietary rehabilitation after 5 months.[13]

López-Santamaría and colleagues[35] described a single case of MVT in a 16-year-old patient with CIPO, who died from MOF 39 days post-transplantation.

In 2006, Takahashi and colleagues[36] published a case of an 8-year-old patient who received an MMVT for CIPO. She suffered recurrent bouts of acute rejection with coexisting chronic rejection and underwent retransplantation of all allografts 250 days after the original operation.

A 2008 case report from the University of California at Los Angeles outlines the course of MVT in a 28-year-old woman with a hypertrophic variant of congenital visceral myopathy who developed CIPO and TPN-induced liver failure after being on lifelong TPN since the age of 2 years. At 2 years post-MVT, she was maintaining her weight on enteral feeds without TPN, pancreatic enzyme replacement, or insulin.[37]

The transplant program at the University of Pittsburgh performed 36 MMVTs at their center between 1990 and 2010, 19 of which were indicated for CIPO secondary to visceral myopathy and/or neuropathy with extensive GI involvement. All patients were on home PN (HPN) and lacked hepatic dysfunction. The technique of preserving the native spleen, pancreas, and duodenum was performed in 16 out of 19 cases, including shortening of the retained duodenum to prevent segmental dysmotility. Three of these patients developed post-transplant allograft dysmotility postoperatively; however, all but 2 patients who underwent MVT for intestinal pseudo-obstruction saw an improvement in dysmotility by a year postoperatively.[12] The cases of MMVTs reported in this study occurred primarily in adults, which is consistent with the increased susceptibility of developing livers to HPN.[6,12]

In a retrospective case review, Mangus and colleagues[6] analyze the cases of MVTs at Indiana University between 2004 and 2010. Seven of 95 patients were presented with pseudo-obstruction during this period, 1 requiring MVT and 6 requiring MMVT. Due to a learning curve for performing these complex operations, the center saw an increase in 3-year patient survival from the period of 2004 to 2007 to the period of 2007 to 2010; survival increased from 44% to 56% for adult recipients of MVT and from 67% to 80% for adult MMVT recipients.[6]

From 2000 to 2011, 2 adults underwent MVT for CIPO at the University of Bologna, while 9 adults underwent isolated intestinal transplant for the same issue. Both patients who received MVT died postoperatively, one from hemolytic uremic syndrome and one from sepsis.[38]

Grosman and colleagues[39] summarize a pediatric case of MVT for CIPO at the age of 5 years. The patient's disease course prior to transplantation was complicated by chronic obstruction requiring TPN, decompression gastrostomy, and ileostomy; recurrent central venous line infections; and hepatic fibrosis. The graft consisted of the liver, stomach, duodenum, pancreas, small bowel, and right colon. He was able to completely wean off TPN by 2 months post-transplantation. Five years after undergoing MVT, the patient is doing well overall and supplements oral intake with gastrostomy tube (G-tube) feedings.[39]

Megacystis microcolon intestinal hypoperistalsis syndrome

Megacystis microcolon intestinal hypoperistalsis syndrome (MMIHS) is a rare autosomal recessive disorder that presents in the neonatal period and is characterized by bowel obstruction in the absence of anatomic obstruction.[40] Though multiple sources describe MMIHS as a congenital form of CIPO, the authors have chosen to list MMIHS as a separate indication for MVT due to its distinguishing clinical features of nonobstructive urinary distension, malrotation, and narrowed distal ileum and colon in addition to the GI hypoperistalsis seen in both CIPO and MMIHS.[34,39,40]

From 1994 to 1998, 3 patients underwent MVT for MMIHS. All 3 patients presented with jaundice and hepatomegaly and had SBS due to a history of multiple bowel resections. All patients were female and were 7.7, 10.3, and 33.1 months of age. Their clinical history included long-term TPN with ensuing liver disease and recurrent urinary tract infections, with 1 patient developing portal hypertension. The patients received en bloc grafts that included the stomach, small bowel, liver, pancreas, and both kidneys. The first 2 recipients also received the large intestine up the transverse colon. Patient 1 died 17 months post-transplantation, from aspiration after revision of her G-tube; at the time of death, she was off TPN. Patient 2 was still alive at 17 months and able to maintain her weight entirely on enteral feedings. Patient 3 developed acute severe rejection of the intestinal graft and died 44 days post-transplantation of multisystem failure secondary to Serratia-induced septic shock.[40]

Loinaz and colleagues published a retrospective review from the same center in 2004 that summarizes 5 additional cases of MVT indicated for MMIHS.[33] The patients were PN-dependent and required MVT for either liver disease, loss of venous access, or sepsis. The 2-year survival rate for all reported cases, including 8 total patients with MMIHS and 8 patients with CIPO, was 42.9% for the period from 1996 to 2000 and

77.8% for the period from 2001 to 2004. All the long-term survivors were able to maintain weight with solely enteral feedings. The same center published a report the following year describing 6 cases of MVT performed for MMIHS; there is likely an overlap between these cases.[33,34]

Nathan and colleagues[41] report 1 case of a patient with MMIHS who underwent MVT at 10 months of age. The patient received a graft consisting of the liver, small bowel, pancreas, and colon and was able to tolerate 100% enteral nutrition.

Tzakis and colleagues[5] report in their single-center review from Miami 7 cases of MVT indicated for MMIHS in pediatric patients.

A 2012 case report from Duke University summarizes the case of a male patient with MMIHS who received an MVT at 22 months of age. He experienced several complications of TPN, including cholestatic liver disease, bacterial and fungal central line infections, and left subclavian vein thrombosis. He received a graft consisting of the liver, small bowel, and pancreas. The patient was able to transition to enteral feeds 4 weeks after surgery, and at his 16-month follow-up, he had yet to experience any major postoperative complications.[42]

Finally, Kunzler and colleagues[43] report a case of MVT for MMIHS in a 12-month-old male. He also had malrotation, intestinal failure–associated liver disease (IFALD), portal hypertension, and bilateral hydronephrosis. He received an en bloc graft that included 2 kidneys, 2 ureters, and a bladder segment containing the vesical trigone. He had normal allograft function at 2 years and 10 months post-transplant.[43]

Hirschsprung disease
Hirschsprung disease, also known as congenital aganglionic megacolon, is a motor disorder of the colon characterized by the failure of neural crest cells to migrate rostrocaudally to the distal colon. Subtypes are classified by the extent of colonic involvement. The predominant type is short-segment Hirschsprung disease, in which only the most distal segment of the rectosigmoid colon is involved. The long-segment variation is characterized by the proximal extension of aganglionosis to the splenic flexure. Total colonic aganglionosis is characterized by full colonic involvement, and the relatively rare total intestinal aganglionosis includes involvement of the small bowel from either the duodenum or the proximal jejunum; this subtype has the highest morbidity and mortality.[44,45]

At the University of Miami between 1994 and 2005, 8 patients (7 children, 1 adult) received MVT for Hirschsprung disease.[5] Takahashi and colleagues[46] published a case of a patient with Hirschsprung disease who underwent MVT at age 6 years and then retransplantation at age 10 years. The original allograft included the stomach, pancreas, duodenum, small intestine, and large intestine. The patient's postoperative course was characterized by chronic rejection, and he was placed on the list for a second MVT. The function of the second graft was normal postoperatively, but the patient died 21 days after the second transplant of suspected rupture of a pseudoaneurysm of a donor abdominal aorta.[46]

Intestinal neuronal dysplasia
Intestinal neuronal dysplasia (IND) is a highly contested topic in the literature. Two types have been described, though type B is more prevalent in the literature due to type A's relative rarity and diagnostic difficulty. Type B is characterized by hyperplasia and dysplasia of the parasympathetic submucosal plexus, resulting in dysfunctional "giant" ganglia, and a presentation similar to Hirschsprung disease.[47]

Loinaz and colleagues[34] report 1 case of a 17-year-old patient undergoing MVT for IND. The fact that IND is a contested diagnosis may be a contributing factor to the dearth of support in the literature for IND as an indication for MVT.

Indication for Multivisceral Transplant: Other Pediatric Conditions

There are also GI pathologies unique to the pediatric population, particularly conditions that are congenital or may present in the neonatal period, that can cause SBS and/or intestinal failure and thus are indications for MVT.

Necrotizing enterocolitis (NEC) is a relatively common life-threatening illness associated with prematurity that frequently becomes a surgical emergency.[48] One case report from the University of Miami discusses a 7-year-old female with SBS due to NEC at age 2 months leading to IFALD. She had a primary MVT at age 6 months with stable graft function in the first year but developed PTLD, had MOF due to sepsis, progressed to end-stage renal disease, and lost the graft due to chronic rejection. However, she had a second MVT at age 7. Due to chronic GVHD, she developed aplastic anemia and required autologous bone marrow transplant of stem cells from the donor. At 5 years post-transplant, she still required recurrent transfusion but was off immunosuppression and had normal allograft function.[43] Three other pediatric patients from the University of Miami also received MVT for SBS secondary to NEC. All patients had intestinal failure and were TPN-dependent. One patient was a male with NEC involving the small bowel and colon who first received a primary intestine-pancreas transplant at age 1.9 years that resulted in severe acute rejection and died 3 months post-transplant due to MOF. Another patient was a female with NEC involving the small bowel and colon who received MVT at age 5.1 years and was alive at the last follow-up 32 months post-transplant. The third patient was a male with NEC involving the small bowel and colon who received MVT at age 9.9 years and was alive at the last follow-up 21 months post-transplant. A multivisceral graft including stomach and pancreas was chosen in these last 2 patients due to severe adhesions in the upper abdomen in 1 case and hemorrhagic pancreatitis in the other. The 2 surviving patients have been weaned off TPN and have functional grafts.[48] Another patient in a different study received MVT for intestinal failure due to NEC but died of cardiopulmonary arrest of unknown etiology 35 days later. This patient was part of a retrospective analysis of patients with intestinal failure and ESLD due to TPN-induced cholestasis who underwent isolated liver transplant (ILT) at Cincinnati Children's Hospital Medical Center.[41]

MVT has also been performed for intestinal failure associated with conditions such as gastroschisis, malrotation, and volvulus. Three other patients in the study from Cincinnati Children's Hospital had MVT for these aforementioned reasons. One patient had intestinal failure due to gastroschisis and midgut volvulus. They received MVT at age 21.6 months but died of recurrent massive upper GI hemorrhage on post-transplant day 56. The second patient had intestinal failure due to gastroschisis and midgut volvulus. This patient died 16.9 months after MVT due to subdural hematoma secondary to nonaccidental trauma but had been TPN-independent with normal serum bilirubin level at the time of death. The third patient had intestinal failure due to malrotation and midgut volvulus. After MVT, this patient eventually became TPN-independent and was alive at the last follow-up. The 4 patients all received liver-small bowel-pancreas allografts. The 2 surviving patients are TPN-independent and have bilirubin levels within the normal range.[41] One patient from a study by Ravindra and colleagues[42] similarly received MVT for intestinal failure secondary to SBS due to gastroschisis, complicated by severe TPN-induced cholestasis. She was weaned off TPN by week 6 and was alive at the 4-month follow-up. Cauley and colleagues[49] presented a case report from Children's Hospital Boston of a 3-month-old premature infant diagnosed with gastroschisis antenatally who suffered midgut volvulus on day of life 2. She developed SBS from extensive bowel resection and PN-associated liver disease.

Interestingly, the investigators specify that MVT, rather than combined liver-intestine transplantation, was performed for technical reasons due to the small size of both the donor (2.9 kg) and the recipient (3.2 kg). This is an important consideration in pediatric, but more specifically neonatal, indications for MVT. Six years later, she had had excellent growth and normal allograft function with no evidence of GVHD.[49] In the review by Tzakis and colleagues,[5] other pediatric indications included gastroschisis (n = 18), NEC (n = 9), intestinal atresia (n = 9), volvulus (n = 4), and microvillous inclusion disease (n = 2).

A case report from La Paz University Hospital in Madrid discusses a rare autosomal recessive condition, Mitchell-Riley syndrome/Martinez-Frias syndrome (MRS/MFS). They report on the first case that was successfully treated with MVT. The patient was a newborn who presented with duodenal and jejunal atresia, midgut malrotation, hypoplastic pancreas, gallbladder agenesis, and neonatal diabetes; this presentation is classic for this syndrome, but the diagnosis was also confirmed via genetic analysis. The patient had severe intestinal failure and was fully dependent on PN, with PN-associated liver disease. Because the patient had most of the GI abnormalities seen in MRS/MFS, was PN-dependent with associated liver disease, and had suffered multiple episodes of central line–associated sepsis, she was chosen for MVT versus an isolated intestinal graft. After more than 10 years of follow-up, she had normal GI, hepatic, and pancreatic function and nutritional autonomy consuming a regular diet. MRS/MFS is usually lethal within the first year of life due to the severity of associated GI, pancreatic, and hepatobiliary conditions, most of which are not amenable to conventional medical and surgical modalities. MVT appears to be a potential new treatment option.[50]

Nathan and colleagues[41] discuss the advantages and disadvantages of TPN in children with intestinal failure and their implications relating to transplantation. TPN prolongs survival and improves prognosis; however, ESLD due to TPN-induced cholestasis (ESLD-TPN) may preclude its use. ESLD-TPN is an indication for ILT or MVT. Once cholestatic, fibrotic liver disease and portal hypertension develop in patients with intestinal failure, and the ability to achieve enteral autonomy is further compromised because of malabsorption, portal hypertensive enteropathy, and GI bleeding. For patients with intestinal failure and ESLD-TPN, liver replacement therapy is needed. Combined liver-small bowel transplantation or MVT is necessary in patients with irreversible intestinal failure.[41]

Indication for Multivisceral Transplant: Other

A subset of the patients in the studies included received MVT for indications not aligning with the previously delineated categories. Among them, a common theme for MVT indication was SBS and/or abdominal adhesions/frozen abdomen or fibrosis but due to other underlying disease processes or unspecified reasons.

In the review from Indiana University, 18 transplants were done for frozen abdomen/catastrophe, a broad category including patients with history of multiple surgeries, previous radiation therapy, severe trauma, and enterocutaneous fistulae. Fourteen adults and 3 pediatric patients received MVT, while 1 patient received MMVT. In this same study, 22 patients received MVT for intestinal failure with cirrhosis for unspecified reasons, and 8 patients received MMVT for intestinal failure alone.[6] In the review from the University of Miami, 1 adult and 1 pediatric patient received MVT for postoperative abdominal fibrosis.[5]

In the study from the University of Pittsburgh, 2 patients had MMVT for extensive abdominal adhesions with gastric dysmotility after multiple abdominal surgeries.[12] One patient in the study from Iran had developed small-bowel insufficiency 3 months after ex vivo resection of pancreatic carcinoma and small-bowel autotransplantation. He died 5 months after MVT.[15] Girlanda and colleagues[51] discuss a case of intestinal failure after surgical resection of pancreatic blastoma involving the SMA and SMV. He required TPN after his primary resection and developed PN-associated liver disease. The distal ileum and ascending colon were resected due to multiple chronic strictures, leaving him with SBS. This patient underwent MVT with kidney transplantation. The patient was disease-free with normal graft function at the 5-year follow-up with no rejection episodes or pancreatoblastoma recurrence.[51]

One patient from the University of Miami received MVT as a rescue procedure after intestinal autotransplant failure.[14] Kunzler and colleagues[43] discuss a pediatric case from the University of Miami of a 3-year-old male with SBS secondary to multiple bowel resections for incarcerated inguinal hernia at age 7 weeks. He progressed to IFALD. He had his first MVT at age 2 years, which was complicated by acute and chronic rejection and multiple episodes of sepsis leading to permanent renal failure and allograft failure. He had a second MVT 1.5 years later. However, he later developed and died from multidrug-resistant Escherichia coli abdominal sepsis and intestinal allograft failure.[43]

Pascher and colleagues[52] discuss a case of MVT for Crohn's disease in detail. This patient had SBS and frozen abdomen due to fistulizing Crohn's disease s/p multiple abdominal operations. She also had TPN-associated progressive liver cirrhosis with severe portal hypertension. She was TPN-independent after 3 weeks and was discharged with excellent graft function 2.5 months post-transplant.[52]

Finally, a unique case from the University Hospital Jena in Jena, Germany, discusses a patient who was ultimately diagnosed with immunoglobulin (Ig) G4–related systemic disease. Abdominal computed tomography showed a large tumor in the mesenteric root with encasement of the suprarenal inferior vena cava and extended portal and mesenteric vein thrombosis. The patient was listed for MVT after reviewing all diagnostic findings, especially given the SMA aneurysm and deterioration of the patient's condition despite corticosteroid therapy. There were no further complications, in particular no episodes of rejections or infections and no renal function impairment. At the 1 year follow-up, the patient was in good clinical condition. This is the first description of IgG4-associated autoimmunopathy as an indication for MVT.[53]

SUMMARY

Our systematic review aimed to comprehensively collect and analyze the existing literature on indications for MVT. Over the last 3 decades, MVT has been applied sporadically due to the procedure's complexity, a steep learning curve, a shortage of experienced and committed surgeons, and the rarity of the conditions. Our review encompassed a total of 44 studies, delving into various indications such as tumors, ischemia, trauma, dysmotility syndromes, and congenital diseases, marking a significant milestone in the systematic exploration of various treatment options. This comprehensive synthesis of knowledge not only advances our understanding of the field but also holds the potential to catalyze future advancements in this critical area of transplantation medicine.

CLINICS CARE POINTS

- MVT or MMVT has been reported in the treatment of patients with nonresectable slow-growing tumors, with local recurrence after failure of conventional medical or surgical therapy, and with intestinal failure due to SBS secondary to previous tumor resections.

- Diffuse PMT, defined as the complete occlusion of the portal system, is one of the most common indications for MVT.
- Severe trauma involving abdominal organs often requires emergency surgical interventions as lifesaving measures. SBS and other complications may result from the primary procedure(s), resulting in the need for MVT.

DISCLOSURE

None.

REFERENCES

1. Starzl TE, Kaupp HA. MASS HOMOTRANSPLANTATION OF ABDOMINAL OR-GANS IN DOGS. Surg Forum 1960;11:28–30.
2. Starzl TE, Rowe MI, Todo S, et al. Transplantation of Multiple Abdominal Viscera. JAMA, J Am Med Assoc 1989;261(10):1449–57.
3. Huard G, Schiano T, Moon J, et al. Choice of Allograft in Patients Requiring Intestinal Transplantation: A Critical Review. Can J Gastroenterol Hepatol 2017;2017: 1069726.
4. Pugliesi R, Dasyam A, Borhani A. Intestinal and Multivisceral Transplantation - ClinicalKey. Published September 2023. Available at: https://www-clinicalkey-com.proxy.cc.uic.edu/#!/content/playContent/1-s2.0-S0033838923001197? returnurl=null&referrer=null. Accessed September 23, 2023.
5. Tzakis AG, Kato T, Levi DM, et al. 100 multivisceral transplants at a single center. Ann Surg 2005;242(4):480–90 [discussion: 491–3].
6. Mangus RS, Tector AJ, Kubal CA, et al. Multivisceral transplantation: expanding indications and improving outcomes. J Gastrointest Surg Off J Soc Surg Aliment Tract 2013;17(1):179–86 [discussion: 186–7].
7. Abdominal organ cluster transplantation for the treatment of upper abdominal malignancies. - PMC. Available at: https://www.ncbi.nlm.nih.gov/pmc/articles/ PMC1358006/. Accessed October 10, 2023.
8. Olausson M, Friman S, Herlenius G, et al. Orthotopic liver or multivisceral transplantation as treatment of metastatic neuroendocrine tumors. Liver Transplant Off Publ Am Assoc Study Liver Dis Int Liver Transplant Soc 2007;13(3):327–33.
9. Chi Z, Mangus RS, Kubal CA, et al. Multivisceral transplant is a viable treatment option for patients with non-resectable intra-abdominal fibromatosis. Clin Transplant 2018;32(3):e13186.
10. Tryphonopoulos P, Weppler D, Levi DM, et al. Transplantation for the treatment of intra-abdominal fibromatosis. Transplant Proc 2005;37(2):1379–80.
11. Janousek L, Novotny R, Kudla M, et al. Familial Adenomatous Polyposis and Desmoid Tumor Treated with Multivisceral Transplantation and Kidney Autotransplantation: Case Report and Literature Review. Case Rep Surg 2019;2019: 6064720.
12. Cruz RJ, Costa G, Bond G, et al. Modified "liver-sparing" multivisceral transplant with preserved native spleen, pancreas, and duodenum: technique and long-term outcome. J Gastrointest Surg Off J Soc Surg Aliment Tract 2010;14(11): 1709–21.
13. Jovine E, Masetti M, Cautero N, et al. Modified multivisceral transplantation without a liver graft for Gardner/Desmoid syndrome and chronic intestinal pseudo-obstruction. Transplant Proc 2002;34(3):911–2.

14. Samuk I, Tekin A, Tryphonopoulos P, et al. Abdominal transplantation for unresectable tumors in children: the zooming out principle. Pediatr Surg Int 2016; 32(4):337–46.
15. Nikeghbalian S, Mehdi SH, Aliakbarian M, et al. Multivisceral and small bowel transplantation at shiraz organ transplant center. Int J Organ Transplant Med 2014;5(2):59–65.
16. Reddy S, Punjala SR, Allan P, et al. First Report With Medium Term Follow Up Of Intestinal Transplantation For Advanced And Recurrent Non-Resectable Pseudomyxoma Peritonei. Ann Surg 2022;277(5):835–40.
17. Vakili K, Kim HB. Partial esophageal transplantation is possible as part of a multivisceral graft. Am J Transplant Off J Am Soc Transplant Am Soc Transpl Surg 2014;14(3):720–3.
18. Clift AK, Giele H, Reddy S, et al. Neoadjuvant peptide receptor radionuclide therapy and modified multivisceral transplantation for an advanced small intestinal neuroendocrine neoplasm: an updated case report. Innov Surg Sci 2017;2(4): 247–53.
19. Moulin L, Rumbo C, Romero P, et al. Case Report: Multivisceral Transplantation for an Extensive Cystic Lymphangioma of the Mesenteric Root. Transplant Proc 2016;48(2):543–5.
20. Olausson M, Friman S, Cahlin C, et al. Indications and results of liver transplantation in patients with neuroendocrine tumors. World J Surg 2002;26(8): 998–1004.
21. Kornberg A, Grube T, Wagner T, et al. Multivisceral transplantation for abdominal malignancy: indication, technique, and results in three patients. Transplant Proc 2001;33(1–2):1558–9.
22. Moulin L, Pedraza N, Padin J, et al. Case Report: Spleen-preserving Multivisceral Transplant for Peutz-Jeghers Syndrome - PubMed. Published March 2016. Available at: https://pubmed.ncbi.nlm.nih.gov/27109998/. Accessed September 28, 2023.
23. Canovai E, Ceulemans L, Gilbo N, et al. Multivisceral Transplantation for Diffuse Portomesenteric Thrombosis: Lessons Learned for Surgical Optimization - PubMed. Published 2021. Available at: https://pubmed.ncbi.nlm.nih.gov/ 33681286/. Accessed September 21, 2023.
24. Vianna RM, Mangus RS, Kubal C, et al. Multivisceral transplantation for diffuse portomesenteric thrombosis. Ann Surg 2012;255(6):1144–50.
25. Florman SS, Fishbein TM, Schiano T, et al. Multivisceral transplantation for portal hypertension and diffuse mesenteric thrombosis caused by protein C deficiency. Transplantation 2002;74(3):406–7.
26. Olausson M, Krantz M, Göthberg G, et al. Multivisceral transplantation in Scandinavia: experiences from the first successful five-organ case. Transplant Proc 2001;33(4):2501–2.
27. Vianna R, Giovanardi RO, Fridell JA, et al. Multivisceral transplantation for diffuse portomesenteric thrombosis in a patient with life-threatening esophagogastroduodenal bleeding. Transplantation 2005;80(4):534–5.
28. Koval CE, Khanna A, Pallotta A, et al. En Bloc Multivisceral and Kidney Transplantation in an HIV Patient: First Case Report. Am J Transplant Off J Am Soc Transplant Am Soc Transpl Surg 2016;16(1):358–63.
29. Nicolau-Raducu R, Livingstone J, Salsamendi J, et al. Visceral arterial embolization prior to multivisceral transplantation in recipient with cirrhosis, extensive portomesenteric thrombosis, and hostile abdomen: Performance and outcome analysis. Clin Transplant 2019;33(8):e13645.

30. Livingstone J, Raveh Y, Souki F, et al. Multivisceral Transplant in a Patient With Portopulmonary Hypertension: A Case Report. Transplant Proc 2022;54(6): 1664–70.

31. Sharkey LM, Russell NK, Rutter CS, et al. Urgent Multivisceral Transplantation for Widespread Splanchnic Ischemia. J Am Coll Surg 2016;222(5):760–5.

32. Nishida S, Hadjis NS, Levi DM, et al. Intestinal and multivisceral transplantation after abdominal trauma. J Trauma 2004;56(2):323–7.

33. Loinaz C, Mittal N, Kato T, et al. Multivisceral transplantation for pediatric intestinal pseudo-obstruction: single center's experience of 16 cases. Transplant Proc 2004;36(2):312–3.

34. Loinaz C, Rodríguez MM, Kato T, et al. Intestinal and multivisceral transplantation in children with severe gastrointestinal dysmotility. J Pediatr Surg 2005;40(10): 1598–604.

35. López-Santamaría M, Gámez M, Murcia J, et al. Intestinal transplantation in children: differences between isolated intestinal and composite grafts. Transplant Proc 2005;37(9):4087–8.

36. Takahashi H, Kato T, Mizutani K, et al. Simultaneous antibody-mediated rejection of multiple allografts in modified multivisceral transplantation. Clin Transpl 2006;529–34.

37. Koh S, Bradley RF, French SW, et al. Congenital visceral myopathy with a predominantly hypertrophic pattern treated by multivisceral transplantation. Hum Pathol 2008;39(6):970–4.

38. Lauro A, Zanfi C, Pellegrini S, et al. Isolated intestinal transplant for chronic intestinal pseudo-obstruction in adults: long-term outcome. Transplant Proc 2013; 45(9):3351–5.

39. Grosman J, Aigrain Y, Goulet O, et al. Preservation of native sigmoid colon for secondary continent cystostomy after multivisceral transplantation for chronic intestinal pseudo-obstruction. Pediatr Transplant 2022;26(2):e14180.

40. Masetti M, Rodriguez MM, Thompson JF, et al. Multivisceral transplantation for megacystis microcolon intestinal hypoperistalsis syndrome. Transplantation 1999;68(2):228–32.

41. Nathan JD, Rudolph JA, Kocoshis SA, et al. Isolated liver and multivisceral transplantation for total parenteral nutrition-related end-stage liver disease. J Pediatr Surg 2007;42(1):143–7.

42. Ravindra KV, Martin AE, Vikraman DS, et al. Use of vascularized posterior rectus sheath allograft in pediatric multivisceral transplantation–report of two cases. Am J Transplant Off J Am Soc Transplant Am Soc Transpl Surg 2012;12(8):2242–6.

43. Kunzler de Oliveira Maia F, Tekin A, Nicolau-Raducu R, et al. Use of pediatric donor en bloc kidneys along with bladder segment in pediatric liver-kidney and multivisceral-kidney transplantation. Pediatr Transplant 2020;24(1):e13596.

44. Chanpong A, Borrelli O, Thapar N. Hirschsprung disease and Paediatric Intestinal Pseudo-obstruction. Best Pract Res Clin Gastroenterol 2022;56-57:101765.

45. Nakamura H, Henderson D, Puri P. A meta-analysis of clinical outcome of intestinal transplantation in patients with total intestinal aganglionosis. Pediatr Surg Int 2017;33(8):837–41.

46. Takahashi H, Delacruz V, Sarwar S, et al. Contemporaneous chronic rejection of multiple allografts with principal pancreatic involvement in modified multivisceral transplantation. Pediatr Transplant 2007;11(4):448–52.

47. Kapur RP, Reyes-Mugica M. Intestinal Neuronal Dysplasia Type B: An Updated Review of a Problematic Diagnosis. Arch Pathol Lab Med 2019;143(2):235–43.

48. Vennarecci G, Kato T, Misiakos EP, et al. Intestinal transplantation for short gut syndrome attributable to necrotizing enterocolitis. Pediatrics 2000;105(2):E25.

49. Cauley RP, Suh MY, Kamin DS, et al. Multivisceral transplantation using a 2.9 kg neonatal donor. Pediatr Transplant 2012;16(8):E379–82.

50. Estefanía-Fernández K, Andrés A, Alcolea A, et al. First multivisceral transplantation in Mitchell-Riley/Martinez-Frias syndrome. Pediatr Transplant 2022;26(5): e14270.

51. Girlanda R, Pozzi A, Matsumoto CS, et al. Multi-Visceral Transplantation in a 21-Year-Old Man with Prior Pancreatoblastoma. Int J Organ Transplant Med 2016; 7(3):193–6.

52. Pascher A, Klupp J, Kohler S, et al. Transplantation of an eight-organ multivisceral graft in a patient with frozen abdomen after complicated Crohn's disease. World J Gastroenterol 2006;12(27):4431–4.

53. Bauschke A, Rauchfuss F, Jandt K, et al. IgG4-related systemic disease–a rare indication for multi-visceral transplantation. Transpl Int Off J Eur Soc Organ Transplant 2012;25(1):e1–4.

Abdominal Wall Closure in Intestinal and Multivisceral Transplantation

A State-Of-The-Art Review of *Vascularized Abdominal Wall* and *Nonvascularized Rectus Fascia* Transplantation

Ewout Muylle, BSc[a,b,c], Nele Van De Winkel, MD[a,d,e],
Ina Hennion, MSc[f], Antoine Dubois, MD[a,b,g], Lieven Thorrez, PhD[f],
Nathalie P. Deferm, MD[h], Jacques Pirenne, MD, PhD[a,b,g],
Laurens J. Ceulemans, MD, PhD[a,c,i],*

KEYWORDS

- Full-thickness abdominal wall transplantation
- Nonvascularized rectus fascia transplantation • Intestinal transplantation
- Multivisceral transplantation • Abdominal wall closure

KEY POINTS

- Abdominal wall closure remains a major surgical challenge with increased morbidity and mortality after intestinal and multivisceral transplantation (Tx) if the abdomen cannot be closed.

Continued

[a] Leuven Intestinal Failure and Transplantation (LIFT) Center, University Hospitals Leuven, Herestraat 49, bus 7003, 3000 Leuven, Belgium; [b] Department of Abdominal Transplant Surgery, University Hospitals Leuven, Leuven, Belgium; [c] Department of Chronic Diseases and Metabolism, Laboratory of Respiratory Diseases and Thoracic Surgery (BREATHE), KU Leuven, Leuven, Belgium; [d] Department of Abdominal Surgery, University Hospitals Leuven, UZ Herestraat 49, bus 7003, 3000 Leuven, Belgium; [e] Department of Development and Regeneration, Unit of Urogenital, Abdominal and Plastic Surgery, KU Leuven, Leuven, Belgium; [f] Tissue Engineering Lab, Department of Development and Regeneration, KU Leuven, KULAK Campus Kortrijk, Etienne Sabbelaan 53, bus 7711, 8500 Kortrijk, Belgium; [g] Department of Microbiology, Immunology and Transplantation, KU Leuven, UZ Herestraat 49, bus 708, 3000 Leuven, Belgium; [h] Department of General and Abdominal Surgery, Sint-Franciscushospital, Pastoor Paquaylaan 129, 3550 Heusden-Zolder, Belgium; [i] Department of Thoracic Surgery, University Hospitals Leuven, Leuven, Belgium
* Corresponding author. Herestraat 49, bus 7003, Leuven 3000, Belgium
E-mail address: laurens.ceulemans@uzleuven.be
Twitter: @CeulemansLJ (L.J.C.)

Gastroenterol Clin N Am 53 (2024) 265–279
https://doi.org/10.1016/j.gtc.2023.12.001

Continued

- Full-thickness abdominal wall Tx is a solution when the complete abdominal wall has to be removed with the potential to be used as an immunologic sentinel marker for the intestinal graft.
- Nonvascularized rectus fascia (NVRF) Tx is an easy-to-use and versatile technique, which can be used to bridge larger fascial defects when standard closure techniques are not sufficient.
- NVRF Tx has very good short-term and long-term outcomes with no additional mortality and low incidence of herniation.
- NVRF Tx has the potential for translation outside the context of solid organ Tx because it has been shown in the preclinical setting that it can safely be used without immunosuppression.

INTRODUCTION

Abdominal wall closure is a critical step after intestinal (ITx) and multivisceral transplantation (MvTx). Failure to close the abdomen increases the risk to develop superficial and deep surgical site infections (SSIs), injury to the transplanted organ and fistulation. This results in an elevated morbidity (50%) and mortality (10%).[1,2] However, closing the abdomen is a challenge due to atrophy, scarring, and muscle retraction of the recipient's abdominal wall as a consequence of previous surgeries and presence of ostomy.[3] Moreover, a large number of these patients have a so-called hostile abdomen originating from earlier infections and abdominal adhesions.[2] This closure challenge is further aggravated by reperfusion edema of the donor organs and recipient.[3] Closure under traction must be avoided because it has the potential to induce abdominal compartment syndrome and graft ischemia.[3–5] Reports indicate that primary closure of the abdominal wall in ITx recipients is achieved in 40% to 85% of cases. However, 20% to 33% of patients who undergo primary closure, experience postoperative wound dehiscence.[6] Additionally, resorting to secondary or staged closure lengthens hospitalization and impedes the overall postoperative recovery process.

To overcome the challenge of abdominal wall closure after ITx and MvTx, numerous techniques have been described, categorizable into 3 primary groups.[7] First, *reduction techniques* involve the reduction of the transplanted organs' size, splenectomy, or selecting a smaller donor than recipient. Second, *expansion techniques* encompass the use of (inflatable) tissue expanders (subcutaneous, intraperitoneal, or retromuscular placement) and secondary or delayed closure.[8] Third, abdominal wall reconstruction and substitution techniques include the application of synthetic, biological, or biosynthetic meshes and autologous tissue transfers (including the use of pedicled or free local flaps).[4,9] However, despite the variability of available methods, each presents limited indications and carries the risk of specific complications.[2] Alternatively, 2 techniques that belong to the latter category are the (full-thickness) abdominal wall vascularized composite allograft (AW-VCA) Tx and the use of nonvascularized rectus fascia (NVRF). Although rarely performed, these techniques prove particularly advantageous in addressing extensive abdominal wall defects.

Clear definition of these reconstruction options is key since they are too often all classified as abdominal wall Tx in literature. Regarding AW-VCA, this involves the Tx of the abdominal wall as a full-thickness vascularized, myocutaneous free flap comprising one or both rectus abdominis muscles with fascia, overlying subcutaneous

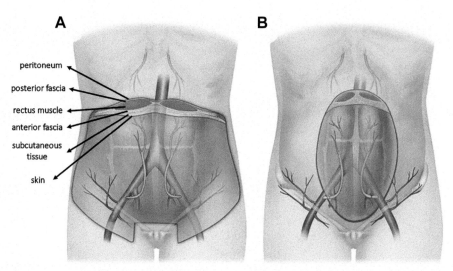

Fig. 1. Layers and blood supply of the full-thickness abdominal wall vascularized composite allograft. (*A*) The full-thickness abdominal wall vascularized composite allograft consists of (from anterior to posterior) skin, subcutaneous tissue, anterior rectus fascia sheet, rectus muscles, posterior rectus fascia sheet and peritoneum. Here, a type of macroanastomosis is illustrated comprising the external iliac and femoral artery cuff (with branches: deep inferior epigastric arteries, deep circumflex iliac artery, superficial circumflex iliac artery, and superficial inferior epigastric artery). (*B*) AW-VCA Tx with the microsurgical technique in which epigastric vessels are anastomosed to provide revascularization. (*Adapted from* Avashia YJ, Mackert GA, May B, Erdmann D, Ravindra K V. Abdominal Wall Transplantation. Curr Transplant Reports. 2015;2(3):269-275. https://doi.org/10.1007/s40472-015-0070-9; with permission)

tissues and skin (**Fig. 1**A).[10] This free flap is transplanted together with its blood supply, mainly provided through the inferior epigastric vessels, which are anastomosed with the recipient's vessels (**Fig. 1**A and B).[9] This technique was introduced by the Miami transplant group in 2003 and several variations of their technique have been proposed since.[10] NVRF Tx entails the Tx of solely the rectus fascia (typically both anterior and posterior rectus sheet) and peritoneum, after the removal of the rectus muscles without any vascular anastomosis (**Fig. 2**).[11] Hence, it could be more accurately described as a type of tissue transfer. This technique was firstly described by Gondolesi and colleagues at Mount Sinai, New York in 2009.[12] A variation of this technique is the use of a vascularized, posterior rectus fascia graft, with blood supply facilitated through the falciform ligament. Consequently, this can only be performed if the liver is included in the transplanted graft. This technique was proposed by Agarwal and colleagues in 2010 and initially described to obtain abdominal wall closure in pediatric double kidney and liver graft recipients.[13,14] All these techniques share a common goal, which is closure of the abdomen and coverage of the transplanted organs.

This review aims to compare the surgical technique, immunology, integration (and neovascularization), clinical outcome, and indications for both AW-VCA and NVRF Tx.

DISCUSSION

Table 1 summarizes the main differences between AW-VCA and NVRF Tx.

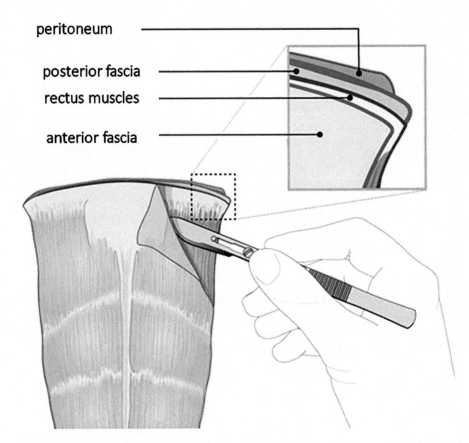

peritoneum

posterior fascia

rectus muscles

anterior fascia

Fig. 2. Layers of the rectus muscle bloc. The rectus bloc consists of (from anterior to posterior) anterior fascia, rectus muscles, posterior fascia and peritoneum. In NVRF Tx, rectus muscles are removed and only both fascia layers and the peritoneum is transplanted.

Surgical Technique

Abdominal wall vascularized composite allograft transplantation

The full-thickness AW-VCA is obtained through a bisubcostal incision that is continued along the lateral edges of the rectus muscles until both groins.[10] For larger defects, a more lateral approach consisting of the external oblique, internal oblique, and transversus abdominis muscles can be included in the graft.[1,15,16] Following, identification of the femoral vessels, a transverse, suprapubic incision is made connecting the incisions on each side.[10] Subsequently, the inferior epigastric vessels are dissected at their origin on the external iliac vessels. The abdominal wall is then flipped over the pubis, packed with cold water and ice and followed by a standard solid organ procurement.[1,10,17] Organ and AW-VCA grafts are flushed and preserved in a cool box. Depending on the chosen anastomosis method, the AW-VCA is excised along with the femoral and iliac vessels, and a short segment of the connecting aorta and inferior vena cava.[10] In the majority of documented cases, both the AW-VCA and the intestinal or multivisceral graft originate from the same donor.

An essential determinant in AW-VCA Tx is providing a reliable vascular supply. Potential recipient vessels for anastomosing an AW-VCA graft are inferior epigastric, deep circumflex, common iliac vessels or infrarenal aorta and vena cava (see **Fig. 1**A and

Table 1
General overview of main differences between full-thickness abdominal wall vascularized composite allograft and nonvascularized rectus fascia transplantation

	AW-VCA Tx	NVRF Tx
General facts		
Graft	Skin Subcutaneous tissue Anterior fascia sheet Rectus muscles Posterior fascia sheet Peritoneum	Anterior fascia sheet Posterior fascia sheet Peritoneum
Vascularization	Revascularization through anastomosis	No need for vascular anastomosis; spontaneous neovascularization
First description	Levi et al. 2003[10]	Gondolesi et al. 2009[12]
Surgical technique		
Incision made for procurement	Bisubcostal, continued along lateral edges and suprapubic incision	Bisubcostal, continued along lateral edges and suprapubic incision
Handling of the vasculature during procurement	Removal of femoral and iliac vessels with short part of the aorta and inferior vena cava together with AW graft (depending on vascular anastomosis technique)	Epigastric vessels are ligated, no large vasculature is included in the graft
Preservation time	Limited to hours	Up to 21 d, possibility for cryopreservation
Use of third-party grafts	Rare	Frequent (1/3)
Immunology		
Need for additional maintenance immunosuppressive drugs	No	No
Immunogenicity	• High; potential use as sentinel marker for cotransplanted intestine • Contributes to differential diagnosis intestinal rejection/infection	• Low (avascular and low cellularity) • Potential formation of fascia-related donor-specific antibodies
Presentation of acute rejection	Nonpruritic, erythematous maculopapular rash on the entire graft, sparing the native skin	Not described
Presentation of GVHD	Generalized rash of the recipient's skin, which is absent on the skin of the AW-VCA	Not described
Integration and neovascularization		
Integration over time	• No spontaneous reinnervation • Hypotrophy of the abdominal wall muscles	• Deposition of collagen around the graft (fibrotic reaction) • Neovascularization => Shown in both experimental and clinical studies

(continued on next page)

Table 1
(continued)

	AW-VCA Tx	NVRF Tx
Clinical experience		
Described cases worldwide	+/− 40	+/− 100
Successful abdominal wall closure	88%	100%
Occurrence of herniation	None	+/− 6%
Patient mortality on the long term (unrelated to abdominal closure)	+/− 50%	+/− 50%
Indication		
	• When the complete abdominal wall is affected and therefore has to be resected • Facilitates primary skin closure	• A more versatile and easy-to-use surgical technique • More suited to be used outside the context of solid organ Tx

B).[9,16,18] Preoperatively visualization of the vascular anatomy of the recipient by CT-scan is therefore essential.[9] Since the initial report, 4 methods for revascularization of the AW-VCA have been described.[1,10,19,20] Levi and colleagues described a macroscopic end-to-side anastomosis of the donor's epigastric vessels of the AW-VCA to the recipient's common iliac vessels or infrarenal aorta and inferior vena cava.[9,10] As demonstrated in cadaveric studies, isolating the iliofemoral cuff pedicle yields in a greater mean area of the abdomen being perfused, than only perfusing the deep inferior epigastric artery.[16] In this technique, microsurgery is not required, although an additional operative time of 2 hours is reported.[9,10] Alternatively, revascularization can be achieved through microanastomosis, initially described by Cipriani and colleagues.[1] In this approach, the inferior epigastric vessels of the donor are sectioned at their origin on the iliac vessels and sutured to the recipient's epigastric or circumflex deep inferior vessels in an end-to-end way with microsurgery using 9-0 Prolene sutures.[1,17] The rationale behind this technique is that iliac vessels of the donor can remain in situ and serve as a vascular graft if needed during the MvTx. The additional operative time of this microsurgical technique was reported to be also 2 hours.[1,17]

In conclusion, a disadvantage of the latter 2 techniques is the prolonged ischemia time because the AW-VCA is transplanted after the already time-consuming solid organ transplantation (SOTx). This may result in increased ischemia-reperfusion injury of the AW-VCA as well as rhabdomyolysis of the transplanted muscle and consequently increased graft failure. Moreover, prolonged ischemia time also increases the risk of sensitization for rejection.[19]

Therefore, Giele and colleagues described a new technique in 2014 designed to enable immediate revascularization of the graft.[19] In this approach, temporary revascularization of the AW-VCA, simultaneously with the solid organ graft, is provided through the ulnar and radial artery of the recipient's forearm. This requires a concomitant operation by the plastic surgery team. After the SOTx has been performed, permanent revascularization of the abdominal wall is established by redirecting the blood supply to the recipient's vessels, if feasible. Although this is an elegant option to reduce ischemia time of the AW-VCA, it adds more complexity to the overall procedure and can lead to increased postoperative and fore-arm morbidity. Furthermore, an additional procedure might be needed.[3,9,19] The most recent approach was introduced by Erdmann and colleagues at Duke University Hospital, involving the creation of a temporary arteriovenous loop with the saphenous vein.[20] Later on, the loop is transected and an anastomosis is made with the inferior epigastric vessels of the donor in an end-to-end way. This technique results in a shorter ischemia time of the AW-VCA and shorter total operative time.[20]

Nonvascularized rectus fascia transplantation

In this technique, only the fascia sheets (anterior and posterior) are transplanted following removal of the rectus muscles. Preserving the internal peritoneal layer is crucial because it helps to prevent the development of abdominal wall adhesions with intra-abdominal content.[3,5] The graft procurement starts with a midline incision up to the anterior sheet of the rectus fascia. The anterior fascia is then completely exposed by lateral dissection toward the oblique muscles (**Fig. 3**A). Subsequently, the rectus muscles, along with fascia sheets and peritoneum, are transected at their cranial insertion on the costal cartilage, followed by bilateral vertical transection of the 3 muscle layers of the lateral abdominal wall. After the organ procurement, the muscle flap is resected (**Fig. 3**B) and, on the bench, the rectus muscles are removed (**Fig. 3**C).[12] Lesions and openings from perforating arteries in both fascial layers are closed with 2-0 polypropylene sutures.[3,21] This also closes the fascial layers preventing large compartments to be filled with fluid, forming seroma. The donor's abdominal cavity is closed using a plastic sheet over which the skin is approximated (**Fig. 3**D). The NVRF graft is stored on ice in preservation solution to which antibiotics can be added (eg, gentamicin), limiting the risk of postoperative SSI. Preservation times up to 21 days have been reported.[5,21] Alternatively, NVRF grafts can be cryopreserved as already performed in a few cases (personal communication with the Miami transplant group).[21] This cryopreservation option allows for prolonged preservation, enabling third-party NVRF Tx (where the NVRF graft comes from a different donor than the solid organ graft). A multicentric, international survey coordinated by our group, comprising 98 cases of NVRF Tx, revealed that approximately one-third of the transplanted NVRF grafts are originating from a third-party donor.[22] The NVRF graft is sutured with continuous or interrupted stitches (Prolene 2/3–0) to the native fascia of the recipient (**Fig. 3**E). In cases where primary closure is not achievable, a vacuum-assisted closure (VAC) device can be placed on top of the fascia, followed by secondary closure (**Fig. 3**F).[3] Covering the NVRF with wet dressings is not recommended due to the increased risk of wound infection.[2]

In contrast to AW-VCA Tx, NVRF Tx does not require vascular anastomosis, limiting additional operative time. Consequently, it is considered a more versatile and easier-to-learn technique.

Immunology

Abdominal wall vascularized composite allograft transplantation

Based on the available experience, no additional maintenance immunosuppressive drugs are required in case of AW-VCA Tx.[9] An acute rejection macroscopically manifests as a nonpruritic, erythematous maculopapular rash on the entire graft, sparing the native skin (**Fig. 4**A). Treatment involves intravenous steroids combined with the topical use of tacrolimus until the rash resolves.[6]

An important aspect is to understand if adding an AW-VCA to an intestinal or multivisceral graft increases the risk of rejection due to the higher antigen load. The skin is recognized as highly immunogenic tissue, given the antigen-presenting capacity of

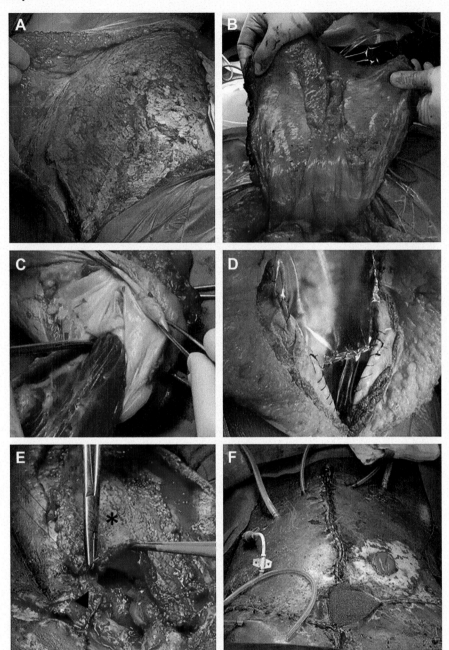

Fig. 3. Surgical technique of NVRF Tx. (*A*) After midline incision up to the anterior sheet of the rectus fascia, a lateral dissection toward the obliques muscle is performed. (*B*) After transection at the cranial insertion of the rectus muscles on the costal cartilage and bilateral vertical transection of the muscle layers of the lateral abdominal wall, the rectus bloc is flipped over and resected and standard organ procurement is performed. (*C*) The rectus muscles are removed from the bloc on the bench. (*D*) The donor's abdominal cavity is closed with a plastic sheet after organ and NVRF procurement. On top of this sheet, the skin is approximated. (*E*) The NVRF graft (*black asterisk*) is sutured to the edges of the native abdominal wall (*black arrow head*) with a continuous suture. (*F*) The skin can be primary closed on top of the NVRF graft. If this is not possible, a VAC-pump can be applied.

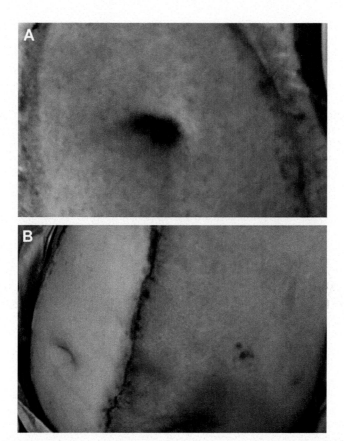

Fig. 4. Presentation of acute rejection and GVHD in the transplanted AW-VCA. (*A*) Clinical presentation of an acute rejection of the AW-VCA after Tx. Rejection presents through a nonpruritic, erythematous maculopapular rash on the entire graft, sparing the native skin. (*B*) Clinical presentation of GVHD in the context of AW-VCA Tx. GVHD presents through generalized rash of the recipient's skin, sparing the AW-VCA's skin. (*Data from* Gerlach UA, Vrakas G, Sawitzki B, et al. Abdominal Wall Transplantation: Skin as a Sentinel Marker for Rejection. Am J Transplant. 2016;16(6):1892-1900. https://doi.org/10.1111/ajt.13693.)

epithelial cells, as they can express class II major histocompatibility complex molecules, particularly during inflammation.[6,23,24] Moreover, epidermal Langerhans cells have the possibility to directly stimulate recipients' T-cells.[6]

The skin of the AW-VCA could function as a sentinel marker for the cotransplanted intestine, offering easy accessibility for monitoring acute rejection. Consequently, the need for intestinal graft biopsies with its associated risks (ulceration and perforation) could be avoided. In addition, rejection of the skin component of the AW-VCA may precede intestinal rejection, providing a certain amount of so-called lead time.[6] However, there are conflicting reports describing the occurrence of isolated rejection of the intestinal graft in absence of AW-VCA rejection or cases where intestinal rejection preceded AW-VCA rejection.[25,26] Another suggested benefit of combined ITx/MvTx and AW-VCA Tx is to help differentiate intestinal rejection and infection, which can present clinically and histologically in a similar manner. In this scenario, antirejection medication could be withheld until microbiological proof is available if no cutaneous rejection signs in the AW-VCA are present: a so-called intention-not-to-treat protocol, proposed by Gerlach and colleagues.[6]

A third immunologic benefit of AW-VCA is its potential protective effect on the solid organ graft. In a cohort study of 28 patients, a lower rate of intestinal graft rejection was observed in patients who had an additional AW-VCA Tx simultaneously with an ITx, whereas the overall survival was equal to patients who only received SOTx.[6] In a retrospective cohort study of 32 patients, Weisenbacher reported no increase in donor-specific antibodies in patients who underwent a combined ITx/MvTx and AW-VCA Tx compared with isolated ITx or MvTx.[27]

Chronic rejection in VCA in general is not well understood. The Oxford group reported one case of chronic rejection.[4] However, consequent fibrotic reaction around the graft might have limited clinical impact, contributing to the strength and coverage of the abdominal wall in the recipient.[26]

In case of graft-versus-host disease (GVHD), the addition of an AW-VCA could facilitate a more rapid diagnosis. In patients without an AW-VCA Tx, GVHD diagnosis may be delayed, presenting with nonspecific skin and gastrointestinal symptoms. GVHD clinically manifests as a generalized rash on the recipient's skin, absent on the skin of the AW-VCA (**Fig. 4**B).

Overall, AW-VCA Tx does not only provide closure of the abdomen but could also serve as an immunologic surrogate for the solid organ graft. However, this experience is based on small patient cohorts, and careful consideration is warranted to weigh this theoretic benefit against the accompanying risks, especially if AW-VCA Tx is not strictly necessary to bridge the recipient's abdominal wall.

Nonvascularized rectus fascia transplantation

Similar to AW-VCA Tx, Tx of NVRF does not require additional immunosuppression. Because an NVRF graft is avascular and has a low cellular density, it is generally considered as nonimmunogenic and consequently ABO-matching and human leukocyte antigen-matching are theoretically not required.[2,21] However, the Cambridge group reported a case of the presence of de-novo donor-specific antibodies against the fascia graft. Furthermore, cases of cytomegalovirus transmission have been documented.[5] In our own experience, we transplanted a non-ABO-matched NVRF (in which an O-recipient received a graft from an A-donor), resulting in elevated natural and immune anti-A antibodies in the recipient's serum 6 days posttransplantation.[28] These cases suggest the occurrence of a host immune response against the transplanted tissue, possibly triggered by the cell-rich composition of the peritoneum.[2]

Understanding this process of immune response against NVRF is also crucial outside the context of SOTx. In preclinical experiments of our group, NVRF allografts were transplanted into 12 rabbits (6 allogeneic and 6 syngeneic rabbits) without immunosuppression. Comprehensive histologic and immunohistochemical analyses were performed 4 weeks after Tx. An inflammatory cell infiltrate was seen consisting of lymphocytes and macrophages (forming foreign body giant cells), particularly at the interface with the native abdominal wall. This infiltrate was more pronounced in the allogeneic group.[29] In other preclinical study by the group of Gondolesi, 18 NVRF Tx were performed in a rat model (9 in syngenic and 9 in allogenic rats), in the absence of any immunosuppressive drug. Here, CD3+ cells were significantly more present in transplanted NVRF grafts of both groups compared with nontransplanted control grafts. There was no significant relative abundance of CD4+ or CD8+ cells.[30,31] The presence of an immune response against NVRF can facilitate its integration into the native abdominal wall by enhancing the fibrotic reaction around the graft, contributing to its intrinsic strength, comparable to AW-VCA, described above.[28]

Integration and Neovascularization

Abdominal wall vascularized composite allograft transplantation

Following AW-VCA Tx, it is anticipated that the rectus muscles of the graft will experience hypotrophy due to the absence of neurotization.[26] Despite this, hernia formation is rare after AW-VCA Tx, suggesting that reinnervation of the abdominal muscles might not be required for proper morphologic integration and a favorable long-term clinical outcome.[26] This raises the question of whether the Tx of the muscular layer provides an additional advantage, given that the transplanted muscles are not functional in conventional Tx techniques that involve only vascular anastomoses. Nevertheless, Gerlach and colleagues reported the recovery of rectus muscle contractility in 3 patients out of a case series of 13 patients. Autonomic functions such as sweating and piloerection were also observed.[6] Surgical technique for isolating the thoracolumbar nerves has been described in cadaveric and animal studies.[9,32] However, neurotization of the abdominal wall graft might not always be feasible in clinical practice because recipients often have already an extensive abdominal surgical history leading to a locally distorted anatomy of the abdominal wall and the associated nerve structures.[9]

Nonvascularized rectus fascia transplantation

In our short-term rabbit experiments, a good macroscopic integration of the NVRF grafts was observed in all animals. Histologic analysis revealed the deposition of newly formed collagen bundles around the grafts. Immunohistochemical analysis for CD31 demonstrated the presence of neovascularization both at the interphase with the native abdominal wall and in the center of the NVRF graft.[29] In the rat model of the Gondolesi group, collagen fibers were present to a 10-fold larger extent in the syngenic and allogenic group compared with control NVRF. Furthermore, neovascularization was seen in all NVRF grafts (although no immunohistochemical analysis of CD31 was performed). No increase in elastic fibers was observed.[30,31]

Virtually all published NVRF patient cohorts reported satisfactory macroscopic integration of the NVRF, as observed radiologically and during reoperation.[2,22] In our own clinical experience of 3 NVRF Tx after ITx or MvTx, biopsies taken at the interphase revealed an intense fibrotic reaction, primarily composed of collagen bundles, around the NVRF graft, conforming its robust integration. This fibrotic reaction enhances the strength of the NVRF because collagen bundles realign to the direction of applied forces. Furthermore, we could prove the neovascularization process in a unique way by cryogenic contrast-enhanced microCT (cryo-CECT) analysis, revealing newly formed vessels running through the NVRF graft (**Fig. 5**). This cryo-CECT analysis unveiled that vessels originated from the native abdominal wall, subcutaneous layer, and peritoneum.[28]

Clinical Experience

Abdominal wall vascularized composite allograft transplantation

Only a small number of transplant centers have experience in AW-VCA Tx. Therefore, this type of Tx has been performed in only a limited number of patients. The primary objective of achieving abdominal wall closure after visceral Tx has been successfully met in the majority of reported cases.[4] A review comprising 35 patients, reported successful abdominal closure in 88% of the cases after AW-VCA Tx with no related mortality.[3,33] In a systematic review by Reed and colleagues comprising 38 full-thickness AW-VCA, 3 cases had immediate loss of the AW-VCA due to graft failure as a consequence of thrombosis.[34] Late AW-VCA graft loss occurs in 2.5% due to chronic rejection.[4] All these cases involved the Tx of a nonreneurotized graft, leading to speculation

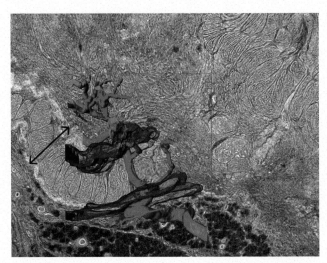

Fig. 5. Cryogenic contrast-enhanced micro-CT analysis of NVRF showing neovascularization. The NVRF graft is indicated with the double black arrow. The 2 blue planes represent the borders of the NVRF graft. One branching blood vessel is reconstructed in red, penetrating the graft.

that patients may develop a large ventral hernia in the long term due to graft atrophy, although such cases have not been explicitly described.[34]

Patients' mortality and solid organ graft loss is not increased after AW-VCA Tx. The reported patient's mortality of 50% is primarily attributed to the cotransplanted intestine, which has its own limitations in terms of outcomes.[4]

Long-term outcome regarding the functionality and influence on the patients' quality of life needs to be addressed in future multicentric studies.[4,34]

Nonvascularized rectus fascia transplantation
Primary closure of the abdominal wall could be achieved in all cases after NVRF Tx.[2,22] In our multicentric, international survey, long-term mortality rate was 51%, which is approximately the same as in AW-VCA Tx. Importantly, this high mortality rate is primarily attributed to the underlying condition of the recipients, particularly in the context of ITx, and not directly related to NVRF Tx. None of the reported mortalities were linked to complications developing from the fascia Tx itself. Initial reports suggested a risk for SSIs in comparison to vascularized rectus fascia Tx, although later publications reported a lower rate of SSIs. In our survey, 31% of the patients experienced an SSI, which is an expected rate in the setting of ITx. We hypothesize that the NVRF graft itself is resistant to SSI. Moreover, NVRF could even be transplanted in the presence of an intra-abdominal infection (and it is considered a preferable option over the use of synthetic meshes in such situations).[5] Moreover, the removal of an NVRF graft is generally not performed due to infection of the NVRF graft. In our international survey, herniation was reported in only 6% of the patients during a median follow-up of 31 months. Furthermore, there was no graft loss reported due to rejection of the NVRF.[22]

Indication

AW-VCA Tx is useful when the complete abdominal wall is affected and therefore has to be resected (eg, due to tumoral processes involving the abdominal wall, extensive scarring, or a complex surgical history). An advantage of this Tx is the facilitation of primary skin closure, given that the graft includes the skin. NVRF Tx is a more versatile surgical technique, particularly suitable for daily clinical practice, especially in addressing large abdominal muscle and fascial defects. NVRF grafts can also be preserved for a long time facilitating its use on demand. Hence, both techniques play valuable roles in distinct surgical contexts. In the near future, both techniques might be used outside the context of SOTx (eg, large herniation defects) in which NVRF Tx seems to be more suited as no additional immunosuppressant drugs are needed.

SUMMARY

Abdominal wall closure after ITx and MvTx remains a challenging problem. In addressing larger defects, Tx of AW-VCA and NVRF have emerged as valuable reconstructive techniques. Both techniques have been proven to be suited in specific indications with a favorable clinical outcome, earning their place in the surgical armamentarium.

CLINICS CARE POINTS

- Obtaining primary closure after ITx or MvTx is essential because failure to do so leads to increased morbidity (with concomitant longer hospital stay) and mortality.
- If the abdominal wall has to be entirely resected or is not sufficient to close the abdomen after SOTx, consider AW-VCA Tx; if only a muscle/fascial defect, consider NVRF Tx.
- Before AW-VCA Tx, imaging of the vascular anatomy in the recipient is essential.
- NVRF Tx is an easy surgical technique in which the graft is not required to be ABO-matched and can be preserved for longer time before Tx.
- When an intra-abdominal infection is present, the use of an NVRF is preferred over the use of a mesh.

ACKNOWLEDGMENTS

The authors thank all members of the Leuven Intestinal Failure and Transplant center. We also thank Dr Cedric Vanluyten for his contribution to the surgical technique figure and Prof Dr Greet Kerckhofs and Arne Maes for providing the figure of the (cryogenic) CECT analysis.

DISCLOSURE

L.J. Ceulemans and L. Thorrez were granted an FTBO grant from KU Leuven; L.J. Ceulemans is appointed as senior clinical investigator for Research Foundation Flanders (FWO).

REFERENCES

1. Cipriani R, Contedini F, Santoli M, et al. Abdominal wall transplantation with microsurgical technique. Am J Transplant 2007;7(5):1304–7.
2. Janssen Y, Van De Winkel N, Pirenne J, et al. Allotransplantation of donor rectus fascia for abdominal wall closure in transplant patients: a systematic review. Transplant Rev 2021;35(4):100634.
3. Fortunato AC, Pinheiro RS, Matsumoto CS, et al. Techniques for Closing the Abdominal Wall in Intestinal and Multivisceral Transplantation: A Systematic Review. Ann Transplant 2022;27:1–14.

4. Honeyman C, Dolan R, Stark H, et al. Abdominal Wall Transplantation: Indications and Outcomes. Curr Transplant Reports 2020;7(4):279–90.
5. Amin I, Canovai E. Closing the abdomen: update on the current surgical toolkit. Curr Opin Organ Transplant 2022;27(2):131–6.
6. Gerlach UA, Vrakas G, Sawitzki B, et al. Abdominal wall transplantation: skin as a sentinel marker for rejection. Am J Transplant 2016;16(6):1892–900.
7. Molitor M, Oliverius M, Sukop A. Abdominal wall allotransplantation. Biomed Pap 2018;162(3):184–9.
8. Ceulemans LJ, Deferm NP, Miserez M, et al. The role of osmotic self-inflatable tissue expanders in intestinal transplant candidates. Transplant Rev 2016;30(4):212–7.
9. Bustos VP, Escandón JM, Santamaría E, et al. Abdominal wall vascularized composite allotransplantation: a scoping review. J Reconstr Microsurg 2022;38(6):481–90.
10. Levi DM, Tzakis AG, Kato T, et al. Transplantation of the abdominal wall. Lancet 2003;361(9376):2173–6.
11. Cassar N, Cortes-Cerisuelo M, Bambridge C, et al. The difficult abdominal closure after paediatric intestinal transplantation: use of abdominal rectus muscle fascia and literature review. Pediatr Transplant 2019;23(5). https://doi.org/10.1111/petr.13473.
12. Gondolesi G, Selvaggi G, Tzakis A, et al. Use of the abdominal rectus fascia as a nonvascularized allograft for abdominal wall closure after liver, intestinal, and multivisceral transplantation. Transplantation 2009;87(12):1884–8.
13. Agarwal S, Dorafshar AH, Harland RC, et al. Liver and vascularized posterior rectus sheath fascia composite tissue allotransplantation. Am J Transplant 2010;10(12):2712–6.
14. Ravindra KV, Martin AE, Vikraman DS, et al. Use of vascularized posterior rectus sheath allograft in pediatric multivisceral transplantation - report of two cases. Am J Transplant 2012;12(8):2242–6.
15. Light D, Kundu N, Djohan R, et al. Total abdominal wall transplantation: an anatomical study and classification system. Plast Reconstr Surg 2017;139(6):1466–73.
16. Hollenbeck ST, Senghaas A, Turley R, et al. The extended abdominal wall flap for transplantation. Transplant Proc 2011;43(5):1701–5.
17. Park SH, Eun SC. Abdominal wall transplant surgery. Exp Clin Transplant 2018;16(6):745–50.
18. Avashia YJ, Mackert GA, May B, et al. Abdominal wall transplantation. Curr Transplant Reports 2015;2(3):269–75.
19. Giele H, Bendon C, Reddy S, et al. Remote revascularization of abdominal wall transplants using the forearm. Am J Transplant 2014;14(6):1410–6.
20. Erdmann D, Atia A, Phillips BT, et al. Small bowel and abdominal wall transplantation: a novel technique for synchronous revascularization. Am J Transplant 2019;19(7):2122–6.
21. Farinelli PA, Rubio JS, Padín JM, et al. Use of nonvascularized abdominal rectus fascia after liver, small bowel, and multiorgan transplantation: long-term follow-up of a single-center series. Transplant Proc 2017;49(8):1810–4.
22. De Winkel N Van, Muylle E, Canovai E, et al. 67: Long-term outcome after non-vascularized rectus fascia transplantation in solid organ transplantation: a global multi-center IRTA survey. Transplantation 2023;107(7S):39.
23. Fan L, Busser BW, Lifsted TQ, et al. Antigen presentation by keratinocytes directs autoimmune skin disease. Proc Natl Acad Sci U S A 2003;100(6):3386–91.

24. Wosen JE, Mukhopadhyay D, MacAubas C, et al. Epithelial MHC class II expression and its role in antigen presentation in the gastrointestinal and respiratory tracts. Front Immunol 2018;9(SEP):408694.
25. Trentadue G, Kats-Ugurlu G, Blokzijl T, et al. Safe and successful treatment of acute cellular rejection of an intestine and abdominal wall transplant with vedolizumab. Transplant Direct 2020;6(2):E527.
26. Selvaggi G, Levi DM, Cipriani R, et al. Abdominal wall transplantation: surgical and immunologic aspects. Transplant Proc 2009;41(2):521–2.
27. Weissenbacher A, Vrakas G, Chen M, et al. De novo donor-specific HLA antibodies after combined intestinal and vascularized composite allotransplantation — a retrospective study. Transpl Int 2018;31(4):398–407.
28. Muylle E, Van De Winkel N, Dubois A, et al. 132: In-depth multi-level analysis of the neovascularization and integration process of a non-vascularized rectus fascia following intestinal transplantation. Transplantation 2023;107(7S):77.
29. Van De Winkel N, Mori Da Cunha M, Pirenne J, et al. OC-009 syngeneic versus allogeneic non-vascularized rectus fascia transplantation in a rabbit model without immunosuppression: short term outcome. Br J Surg 2022;109(Supplement_7). https://doi.org/10.1093/bjs/znac308.021.
30. Moreira J, Stringa P, Gentilini V, et al. 427.6: transplant of the abdominal rectus fascia in rodents, first report of the microsurgical procedure, and initial results. Transplantation 2022;106(9S):S497.
31. Moreira J, Stringa P, Gentilini MV, et al. 42: Early tissue modifications observed in a non immunosuppressed rat model of abdominal rectus fascia transplant. Transplantation 2023;107(7S):23.
32. Broyles JM, Sarhane KA, Tuffaha SH, et al. Reconstruction of large abdominal wall defects using neurotized vascular composite allografts. In: Plastic and reconstructive surgery136. Lippincott Williams and Wilkins; 2015. p. 728–37. https://doi.org/10.1097/PRS.0000000000001584.
33. Berli JU, Broyles JM, Lough D, et al. Current concepts and systematic review of vascularized composite allotransplantation of the abdominal wall. Clin Transplant 2013;27(6):781–9.
34. Reed LT, Echternacht SR, Shanmugarajah K, et al. Twenty years of abdominal wall allotransplantation: a systematic review of the short-and long-term outcomes. Plast Reconstr Surg 2022;150(5):1062E–70E.

Intestinal Transplantation
Include the Spleen with Intestinal Graft?

Rei Matsumoto, MD, PhD, Tomoaki Kato, MD, MBA*

KEYWORDS

- Multivisceral transplant • Acute cellular rejection • Antibody-mediated rejection
- GVHD • Spleen transplantation • Transplant immunology

KEY POINTS

- Including spleen with intestinal graft may increase rejection-free survival time and could potentially decrease the incident rate of severe rejection episodes.
- Including spleen could also normalize the blood cell count and provide protection against encapsuled bacteria.
- There may be a possibility that reperfusion with the donor spleen decreases the level of donor-specific antibody in highly sensitized recipients.
- However, graft-versus-host disease may increase, and the inclusion of the spleen increased autoimmune hemolysis in previous experience.
- The best use of spleen in multivisceral transplant may be to reperfuse with spleen and remove it later.

INTRODUCTION

Outcomes for multivisceral transplantation (MVT) have been improving significantly during the past few years,[1,2] and it has evolved to established therapeutic modality for irreversible intestinal and liver failure. However, since intestine is the most immunogenic of all the solid transplantable organs and have large amount of lymphatic tissue present in the graft, higher incidence rate of rejection and graft-versus-host diseases (GVHDs) have been observed when compared with other solid abdominal organ transplantation.[1,3] Posttransplant infection has been an issue as well; sepsis/infection remains the leading cause of death for intestinal transplant recipients; and using data from ITR, Raghu and colleagues reported that it accounted for nearly half of pediatric patient deaths from 2011 to 2015.[4]

The traditional procedure for MVT is to transplant the stomach, pancreas, intestine, and liver en bloc. During surgery, the native spleen is routinely removed from the recipient, and it usually creates more space in the abdomen to insert the allogeneic graft. Thus, recipients often become asplenic after MVT. There has been an attempt to

Center for Liver Disease and Transplantation, Columbia University Irving Medical Center
* Corresponding author. 622 West 168th Street PH14-105, New York, NY 10032-3723.
E-mail address: tk2388@columbia.edu

gastro.theclinics.com

preserve native spleen in multiviseral cases; however, it has not been incorporated in practice in most places (ref). The spleen is the largest secondary lymphoid organ in the body and hosts wide range of immunologic functions alongside its role as a primary site of blood filtration and hematopoiesis.[5] Asplenic patients are known to be at higher risk of infection by encapsulated bacteria and thrombocytosis.[6]

Because MVT recipients are exposed to higher risk of rejection, GVHD, and infection, inclusion of spleen in the allograft for MVT has been discussed.

ROLE OF SPLEEN IN TRANSPLANTATION IMMUNOLOGY

It is a well-known fact that splenectomized patients are at greater risk of meningitis or sepsis after infection with Streptococcus pneumoniae, Neisseria meningitidis, and Haemophilus influenza type B.[7] These encapsulated bacteria resist the aim of complement immune response of membrane attack complex and can only be responded by the marginal zone macrophages in the spleen.[8]

The spleen's histologic structure is unique and forms the spleen's framework as a blood filter.[8] The spleen is divided by function and structure into the red pulp and white pulp. White pulp of the spleen is a rich reservoir for macrophages, T lymphocytes, and B lymphocytes. The red pulp is composed of a complex meshwork of sinusoids. Blood components flow freely between these red and white pulps and the wide gap between them acts as a filter; the physical organization of the spleen allows it to filter pathogens and abnormal cells and facilitate interactions between antigen-presenting cells and cognate lymphocytes. It is important to note that donor-specific antibodies (DSAs) are reported to be removed effectively through this spleen's filtration by temporary implanting allograft spleen.[9,10]

Native spleen is reported to be a major site for inducing organ rejection. Donor or recipient-derived dendritic cells migrate to spleen and effectively stimulate recipient T cells by presenting alloantigen, which can induce acute rejection.[11] Fabre and colleagues showed that splenectomized rats had longer acceptance of their renal allografts.[12] Furthermore, Blanchard and Tauber reported that when the recipient rats were splenectomized and received donor spleen with the heart, the heart graft survival was prolonged.[13,14] There are other studies showing that the allogenic spleen can also induce donor-specific tolerance to the skin and pancreas.[15,16]

Recent studies have shown that spleen macrophages internalize and remove allogenic T cells.[17] Stringa and colleagues demonstrated in MVT rat models that donor T cell frequency in the bloodstream and skin was significantly reduced when the recipient's spleen was preserved. They also showed that spleen macrophages have the ability to engulf donor T cells in cell transference experiment using fluorescently labeled T cells.[17] However, Fu and colleagues have demonstrated that the donor T cell macrochimerism induced by multiviseral transplant with recipient splenectomy could confer protective effect on intestinal allograft through lymphohematopoietic graft-versus-host reaction (graft-versus-host responses confined to the lymphohematopoietic system) without GVHD.[18]

These reports indicate that spleen is an important site for pathogen or DSA clearance and plays a significant role in cellular-mediated and antibody-mediated rejections. Recent reports also suggest that spleen could reduce allogenic immune cells, which could result in reduced GVHD.

INCLUDING ALLOGRAFT SPLEEN IN MULTIVISCERAL TRANSPLANT GRAFT

In 2007, Kato and colleagues performed a study comparing multivisceral recipients who received a donor spleen (n = 60) with those who did not receive a spleen (n = 81) during the time period of 2001 to 2007.[19,20] In this study, 51 patients in the spleen group received MVT and 9 had modified multivisceral transplant (MMV, MVT without liver). Sixty-eight patients in the control group received MVT and 13 received MMV. There were 49 adults and 92 children in the entire cohort, and children were more likely to have received a spleen. There was no significant difference in patient and graft survival between the spleen and control groups (P = .77 and P = .95, respectively; **Fig. 1**). Average posttransplant white blood cell counts and platelet counts were significantly decreased in spleen group showing its function in normalizing recipient peripheral blood cell counts. Spleen group recipients showed significant superiority in freedom from rejection (P = .02; **Fig. 2**). Inclusion of spleen was also a significant factor favorably associated with freedom from moderate or severe rejection in univariate analysis (P = .02). Analysis of children less than 1 who were transplanted since 2001 revealed that patients in the spleen group showed significantly improved freedom from death due to rejection (P = .03). Incidence of GVHD was 8.25% in the spleen group and 6.2% in the control group, which the difference was not statistically significant (P = .62). This study demonstrated that including spleen in the graft for MVT will not only avoid patients from being asplenic and vulnerable to infection or thrombocytosis but also provide additional protective effect on small bowel rejection without significantly increasing the risk of GVHD. However, subsequent study from the same group showed that the inclusion of the spleen was significant predictor of GVHD.[20] In addition, inclusion of spleen in the allograft was associated with an increased incidence of autoimmune hemolysis. Thus, this practice has been abandoned.

This has prompted some groups to study temporary transplant of the donor spleen; they would transplant the donor spleen with the intestinal allograft, and would subsequently do splenectomy after reperfusion for certain amount of time. Farmer and colleagues investigated factors associated with favorable survival by analyzing 106 intestinal transplantation that was performed between 1991 and 2010.[21] Twenty-four percent of patients underwent recipient splenectomy; 66.7% of donor spleen was removed before transplant and 33.3% was removed after reperfusion for at least an hour. They reported that on univariate analysis, reperfusion of the donor spleen was associated with an improved graft survival, although this was not an independent predictor of survival.

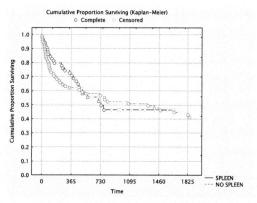

Fig. 1. Patient survival rate of group with spleen and group without spleen transplantation. (*From* Kato T et al. "Transplantation of the Spleen. Effect of Splenic Allograft in Human Multivisceral Transplantation." Annals of Surgery. 2007; 246(3): 436-446; with permission.)

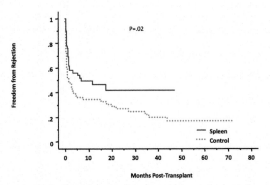

Fig. 2. Freedom from intestinal graft rejection in spleen and control group. (*From* Kato T et al. "Transplantation of the Spleen. Effect of Splenic Allograft in Human Multivisceral Transplantation." Annals of Surgery. 2007; 246(3): 436-446; with permission.)

Temporary transplant of the donor spleen has been studied in other groups as well. Spaggiari has recently published a case report in which a patient received a T-cell and B-cell flow cross-match (FXM) and complement-dependent cytotoxicity cross-match positive intestinal transplant in the presence of several class 1 and 2 DSAs.[9] The patient underwent a "temporary desensitization" using the donor spleen; the deceased-donor spleen was transplanted for an hour and 15 minutes and was removed before transplanting the intestinal graft. They reported significant decrease in class I DSA mean fluorescence intensity in the immediate postsplenic transplant serum resulting in a T-cell negative FXM. Decreased mean channel shift of the positive B-cell FXM was also observed. The explanted splenic allograft showed histopathologic changes that reflect the acute exposure to numerous DSAs; numerous macrophages and neutrophils infiltrated splenic sinusoids and antigen–antibody reaction and complement activation were demonstrated by the diffuse positivity of immunoglobulin G and cluster of differentiation (Cd4) immunohistochemical stains. Spaggiari and colleagues conclude that temporary deceased donor spleen transplantation may play a role in decreasing the risks of rejection in highly sensitized intestinal transplant recipients.

PRESERVATION OF RECIPIENT'S NATIVE SPLEEN

GVHD is feared in intestinal transplantation because large amount of donor lymph tissue will be transplanted together with the intestine. Moreover, transplanting donor's spleen will expose recipients to a higher load of donor's lymphoid tissue. Hence, some groups have been trialing preservation of recipient's spleen in MVT procedures.

Cruz and colleagues reported that preservation of native spleen in modified MVT (MVT sparing liver) was associated with an increased survival and reduced risk of GVHD and posttransplant lymphoproliferative disorders (PTLDs).[22] They investigated 36 modified MVT cases in which spleen was preserved in 24 cases. Incidence rate of acute intestinal allograft rejection was not significantly different between the group that underwent major evisceration technique and spleen preservation group (58% and 63%, respectively; $P = .139$). However, incidence rate of severe rejection was higher in spleen preservation group (14% and 60%, respectively; $P = .057$). They observed GVHD in 25% of splenectomy group; however, no GVHD was diagnosed in spleen-preserved group.

Stringa and colleagues compared 81 patients (51 patients received isolated small bowel transplant, 24 received MVT, and 6 received liver and intestinal transplantation) that underwent spleen preservation to 42 patients (1 patient received isolated small bowel transplant, 24 received MVT, and 17 received liver and intestinal transplantation) that underwent splenectomy and 14 patients that underwent allogenic spleen transplantation.[17] They reported that survival rate was significantly better in the spleen preservation group than in the nonspleen or allogeneic spleen groups (66%, 43%, and 34%, respectively; P < .001). No difference in the acute rejection rate was observed; however, although most of the patients in the native spleen preservation and non-spleen groups that developed acute cellular rejection experienced severe episodes, only small portion of allogenic spleen group had severe rejection. The GVHD incidence was significantly lower in the spleen preservation group than in the allogenic spleen group (5% and 43%, respectively; P < .001). They also used rat models to demonstrate that donor T cell frequency in the bloodstream and skin was significantly reduced when the native spleen was preserved. In conclusion, they report that preservation of recipient spleen will significantly decrease circulating donor T cells.

Hernandez and colleagues analyzed 24 MVT cases in which 3 cases underwent spleen preservation.[6] They reported that none of these 3 cases developed GVHD or PTLD while the overall incident rate was 10% and 11%, respectively.

These studies do admit that only selected cases could go through spleen preservation procedure; spleen preservation was abandoned in cases where severe adhesions or inflammation was observed in the pancreatic area or when any damage of the spleen during the manipulation was suspected. Patients with Gardner syndrome often had involvement of the splenic hilum and pancreaticoduodenal complex with desmoid tumors, which precluded them from spleen preservation technique.[22]

DISCUSSION

Outcomes for intestinal transplant and posttransplant quality of life have been improving significantly during the past few years; these results indicate that intestinal transplant has clearly been establishing its role as a therapeutic modality for irreversible intestinal failure.

However, the balance between preventing allograft rejection and GVHD has always been a major challenge in postoperative management of intestinal transplant. This is due to intestine being an immunologically complex environment with 80% of immune cells residing within the gastrointestinal system, making the intestine highly immunogenic graft and also exposing the recipient with higher risk of GVHD.

Debate among splenectomy, native spleen preservation, and donor spleen transplantation in MVT has the same logic; it is about the balance of amount and function between donor and recipient's immune cells.

By preserving spleen, immunosuppressed MVT recipients may benefit from spleen's ability to filter pathogens and protect human body from encapsuled bacteria. There are also reports of significant decrease in GVHD incidence rate when native spleen was preserved.[6,17,22] These studies implicated that preservation of native spleen lead to decrease in circulating donor T cells and thus decreased GVHD risk. However, recent study from our institute showed that high levels of peripheral blood T cell mixed chimerism (donor T cell macrochimerism >4%) occur without GVHD in intestinal transplant recipients who underwent splenectomy and are associated with significantly reduced graft rejection,[18] indicating that the presence of circulating donor T cells could be beneficial in protecting transplanted intestinal allograft from host-versus-graft response without initiating graft-versus-host response. Moreover, studies both from spleen preservation and donor spleen transplantation have shown that the presence of native spleen are more likely to induce severe intestinal allograft rejection episodes compared with patients that underwent splenectomy. These results suggest that risk of increasing incidence rate of severe rejection might outweigh the benefit of preserving native spleen. We also have to consider that not all MVT cases are applicable for spleen preservation procedures; only selected cases can be done due to surgical technique limitation and state of recipient's primary disease.

Multiple reports suggested that transplanted allogenic spleen could decrease the incidence rate of severe rejection. However, spleen transplantation significantly increased incidence rate of GVHD and autoimmune hemolysis compared with group that underwent splenectomy. Spaggiari and colleagues reported that even temporary reperfusion of donor spleen could filter and decrease level of circulating DSA level.[9]

Considering all of the risks and benefits, we advocate that temporary transplant of the donor spleen (splenectomy following reperfusion of the donor spleen for a certain amount of time) could be the best option for MVT recipients; it could potentially reduce the rate of intestinal allograft rejection without increasing the risk for GVHD.

Further multivariate analysis with multicenter collaboration needs to be done in which splenectomy, native spleen preservation, and temporary spleen transplantation are directly compared for outcomes, such as rejection rate, infection rate, and GVHD rate.

SUMMARY

The traditional procedure for MVT is to transplant the stomach, pancreas, intestine, and liver en bloc. During surgery, the native spleen is routinely removed from the recipient, both to minimize bleeding and to gain space to insert the allogeneic graft. Spleen is known to play an important role in both innate and adaptive immune responses. It is also a primary site of blood filtration and hematopoiesis. Kato and colleagues compared multivisceral recipients who received a donor spleen (n = 60) with those who did not receive a spleen (n = 81). They demonstrated that including spleen in the graft for MVT significantly increased rejection-free time and significantly decreased death due to rejection in pediatric patients when compared with MVT cases with splenectomy. However, subsequent study from the same group showed that the inclusion of the spleen was significant predictor of GVHD.[20] In addition, inclusion of spleen in the allograft was associated with an increased incidence of autoimmune hemolysis. This has prompted several groups to investigate temporary spleen transplantation, in which donor spleen is implanted with the intestinal allograft and is taken out after reperfusion; by taking it out after reperfusion, it will not increase the risk for GVHD. They have reported that reperfusion of the donor's spleen will significantly decrease the level of DSA in highly sensitized patients. We advocate for temporary spleen transplantation to be more investigated and to be considered as an option for MVT recipients.

CLINICS CARE POINTS

- Including spleen in the graft of MVT could significantly increase the risk of GVHD and autoimmune hemolysis.
- Highly sensitized patients may benefit with spleen transplantation:donor spleen is reported to filter and decrease level of preformed DSAs immediately afer reperfusion.
- Consider temoporary spleen transplantation when performing MVT.

DISCLOSURE

The authors declare no conflicts of interest.

REFERENCES

1. Bhamidimarri KR, Beduschi T, Vianna R, et al. Multivisceral Transplantation Where Do We Stand? Clin Liver Dis 2014;18:661–74.
2. Kaufman SS, Avitzur Y, Beath SV, et al. New insights into the indications for intestinal transplantation: consensus in the year 2019. Transplantation 2020;104(5): 937–46.
3. Andres AM, Ramos E, Hernandez F. Current status of pediatric intestinal transplant in Europe. Curr Opin Organ Transplant 2020;25:183–8.
4. Raghu VK, Beaumont JL, Everly MJ, et al. Pediatric intestinal transplantation: analysis of the intestinal transplant registry. Pediatr Transplant 2019;23(8): e13580.
5. Lewis SM, Williams A, Eisenbarth SC. Structure and function of the immune system in the spleen. Science Immunology 2019;4:eaau6085.
6. Hernandez F, Andres AM, Encinas JL, et al. Preservation of the native spleen in multivisceral transplantation. Pediatr Transplant 2013;17:556–60.
7. Bronte V, Pittet MJ. The spleen in local and systemic regulation of immunity. Immunity 2013;39:806–18.
8. Aliyu M, Zohora F, Saboor-Yaraghi AA. Spleen in innate and adaptive immunity regulation. Allerg Immunol (Leipz) 2020;5(1):1–17.
9. Spaggiari M, Lichvar A, Tzvetanov I, et al. Temporary Deceased Donor Splenic Transplant Prior to Intestinal Transplantation: A New Strategy for Desensitization? Transplant Proc 2021;53:2602–8.
10. Gaitonde S, Hassan M, Mehta V, et al. Histopathology of Human Donor Spleen Utilized as a Desensitization Tool Before Intestinal Transplantation. Am J Clin Pathol 2021;155:621–6.
11. Hara M, Chosa E, Onitsuka T. The spleen's role in transplantation immunology. Transpl Immunol 2008;18:324–9.
12. Fabre JW, Batchelor JR. The role of the spleen in the rejection and enhancement of renal allografts in the rat. Transplantation 1974;17(3):317–9.
13. Blanchard JM, Tauber JW. Heart and spleen twin grafts in rats. J Microsurg 1980; 1(5):381–6.
14. Tauber JW, Blanchard JM. Heart and spleen twin grafts in rats. Delayed host splenectomy. J Microsurg 1981;2(4):261–8.
15. Bitter-Suermann H. Prolonged survival of auziliary spleen allografts in rats inducing acceptance of skin allografts. Transplantation 1974;17:75–83.
16. Bitter-Suermann H, Save-Soderbergh J. The course of pancreas allografts in rats conditioned by spleen allografts. Transplantation 1978;26:28–34.
17. Stringa P, Papa-Gobbi R, Vela M, et al. Native Spleen Preservation During Visceral Transplantation Inhibits Graft-Versus-Host-Disease Development. Clinical and Experimental Study. Ann Surg 2023;277:e235–44.
18. Fu J, Zuber J, Shonts B, et al. Lymphohematopoietic graft-versus-host responses promote mixed chimerism in patients receiving intestinal transplantation. J Clin Invest 2021;131(8):e141698.
19. Kato t, Kleiner G, David A, et al. Inclusion of Spleen in Pediatric Multivisceral Transplantation. Transplant Proc 2006;38:1709–10.

20. Kato T, Tzakis AG, Selvaggi G, et al. Transplantation of the Spleen. Effect of Splenic Allograft in Human Multivisceral Transplantation. Ann Surg 2007;246(3): 436–46.
21. Farmer DG, Venick RS, Colangelo J, et al. Pretransplant Predictors of Survival After Intestinal Transplantation: Analysis of a Single-Center Experience of More Than 100 Transplants. Transplantation 2010;90:1574–80.
22. Cruz RJ, Costa G, Bond G, et al. Modified "Liver-Sparing" Multivisceral Transplant with Preserved Native Spleen, Pancreas, and Duodenum: Technique and Long-Term Outcome. J Gastrointest Surg 2010;14:1709–21.

Intestinal Transplant for Hirschsprung's Disease
Stoma for Life or Not?

Geoffrey James Bond, MD

KEYWORDS

- Hirschsprung's disease • Intestinal transplantation • Pull through procedure
- Intestinal transplant stoma

KEY POINTS

- Intestinal transplants can be performed for Hirschsprung's disease.
- Pull-through procedures in non-transplant patients have complications even after technically excellent operations.
- Intestinal transplants have associated risks related to rejection and immunosuppression but can be managed.
- Pull through of the intestinal allograft can be safely performed.
- Stoma takedown in intestinal transplant recipients can be routinely performed.

INTRODUCTION

Hirschsprung's disease (HD) is a condition where pathologically there is a lack of ganglion cells in the bowel wall that causes dysmotility of the affected bowel. It can occur along varying lengths of the bowel starting most commonly in the distal bowel (rectum and sigmoid colon), but can extend all the way proximally to the upper gastrointestinal (GI) tract in rare cases. The majority of cases can be managed with standard pediatric surgical operations which removes the dysmotile bowel, that otherwise causes a functional obstruction, and brings ganglionated bowel from above this level down to the anorectum to restore continuity of the GI tract. In that way, patients can become enterally independent, and no stoma is required long term. Even after an excellent operative intervention, the condition is not without its own set of short-term and long-term complications. In the very small subgroup of patients with HD where the functional bowel length is so short and reconnection distally is not considered possible, a stoma is brought out, and frequently these patients will need parenteral nutrition (PN) for caloric and fluid support.

Surgical Director, ICARE Children's Hospital of Pittsburgh of UPMC, 4401 Penn Avenue, 6FP Pittsburgh, PA 15224, USA
E-mail address: bondgj@upmc.edu

Gastroenterol Clin N Am 53 (2024) 289–297
https://doi.org/10.1016/j.gtc.2024.03.002
0889-8553/24/© 2024 Elsevier Inc. All rights reserved.

Intestinal transplantation (ITx) is the ultimate therapy for patients with irreversible intestinal failure (IF) and savior for patients that are suffering terminal complications of PN therapy. Over the last 35 years, ITx has become a recognized alternative to lifelong PN therapy, especially when complications have developed. ITx is unlike any other surgical operation in that conceptually it is not a onetime procedure, but a lifelong commitment to maintenance of the allograft through immunosuppression whilst balancing the risks and complications related to the transplanted allograft and the immunosuppression requirements.

In most cases of ITx, there is normally at least some functional GI tract distally that the allograft can be connected to, so as to reestablish intestinal continuity. There may be a proximal diverting stoma temporarily, either to protect the lower anastomosis while it heals and/or to allow for surveillance scoping and biopsies of the allograft, but later this can routinely be taken down and full intestinal continuity can be restored. However, in HD, the distal bowel is dysmotile and unable to be anastomosed to in a standard way, so often no attempt is made to reconnect distally, and a permanent end allograft stoma is made. To perform a reconnection distally, it would need to be a very low bowel anastomosis, and some form of more complicated and potentially risky pull-through procedure (**Fig. 1**) or ileoanal/J pouch procedure is required to establish intestinal continuity. However, if successfully performed, the stoma can then at some point in time be reversed.

Hence the concern and question become should a pull-through procedure, understanding the inherent risks of the procedure in a non-transplant patient, be performed using transplant intestinal allograft. The recipient will still likely have the inherent short-term and long-term concerns seen in non-transplant patients, but additionally and

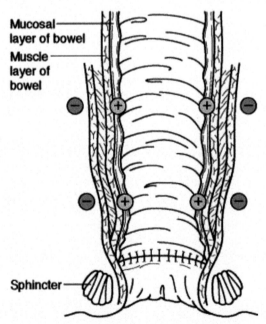

Fig. 1. Soave pull through with the allograft colon (or ileum) being pulled through the muscular cuff and anastomosed to very short segment of native rectum. (*Adapted from* Dasgupta R, Langer JC. Hirschsprung disease. Curr Probl Surg. 2004 Dec;41(12):942-88. https://doi.org/10.1067/j.cpsurg.2004.09.004.

more importantly due to the fact it is allograft bowel, there are added risks of complications such as acute or chronic rejection that could affect the integrity of the low anastomosis and potential impaired healing due to the immunosuppressive medications the recipient is receiving. If it is felt this procedure can safely happen, and be successful, then it would mean the allograft stoma could be taken down and the recipient placed into continuity of the GI tract. If not, then an end stoma would be maintained for life.

This topic was debated at the recent Congress of the Intestinal Rehabilitation and Transplant Association (CIRTA) meeting in July 2023. The following are the key considerations and then review of the somewhat limited experience and literature that went into the final voting process.

SPECTRUM OF HIRSCHSPRUNG'S DISEASE

The vast majority of patients, approximately 85% cases, who have HD fall into the classic variant where the aganglionic distribution is rectosigmoid, and thus a relatively short aganglionic segment. For these cases, multiple different procedures can be done, including the 1-stage neonatal transanal approach or a 1-stage pull through procedure, where no stoma is formed. In other cases, staging is done to determine the level of aganglionosis (leveling procedure), and a diverting stoma brought out. A definitive pull-through procedure is then done either as a 2-stage or 3-stage procedure, where in the end the stoma is taken down completely. There are a number of different pull-through procedures described, and the type used is often up to the surgeon's experience and preference, but this is mostly outside the purvey of this article.

Longer segment HD includes total colonic HD, roughly 10% of cases with HD. These can still mostly be managed with a pull-through procedure or a J pouch/ileoanal procedure as there is sufficient small bowel length for the patient to become enterally independent. Often there may be a temporary stoma, but almost always, these can be reversed.

Total aganglionosis (TAG) or near TAG (NTAG) is seen in less than 5% of cases, with some investigators quoting an incidence as low as 1%. It is thought that approximately 20 to 40 cm of ganglionated bowel is needed to avoid IF. Over time, this short segment will grow in length as the child develops, and other medical strategies (GLP-2 agonist) and pediatric surgical procedures (intestinal-lengthening procedures) may be utilized to get the patient off PN. Whether a permanent stoma is needed, or a reconnection eventually preformed, is dependent on many patient factors. Overall, the number of cases with HD that become permanently PN dependent is very low, the tip of the iceberg so to say, and hence those considered for ITx are rare.

HIRSCHSPRUNG'S DISEASE—POSTOPERATIVE ISSUES

Before addressing ITx for HD, it is important to understand the natural history and known complications of HD both preoperatively and postoperatively. Even after a technically excellent pull-through procedure, there are known frequent complications including incontinence, constipation, enterocolitis, strictures, and transanal prolapse. As well, there are the myriad of stomal issues including stenosis, prolapse, bleeding, skin-related, and stoma appliance–related complications. Hence it needs to be remembered when comparing other therapeutic options, such as ITx, that this is the "baseline" for patients with HD. There is still a lot to be known about HD and the supposedly "unaffected" bowel, such as skip lesions and dysmotility problems, and why postoperative issues arise with the "normal" ganglionated bowel. In fact, it is interesting to hypothesize what would be the result if the "unaffected" bowel were not present and replaced with transplanted intestine, and would this in fact lessen some of the postoperative complications seen such as enterocolitis.

EXTENSIVE HIRSCHSPRUNG'S DISEASE

In patients with extensive HD, autologous intestinal rehabilitation has not overall been successful in helping patients to become enterally autonomous. Such procedures include the Kimura procedure, myectomy/myotomy, skipped aganglionic lengthening transposition procedure, and Lester Martin–modified Duhamel, although these are undergoing further review and consideration. These patients have essentially "short gut syndrome" (SGS), whether anatomically or functionally, and defined as having IF due to inability to absorb enough calories or fluids through their own gut, necessitating PN. As wonderful a treatment PN is for those with IF, it is not without its own set of life-threatening complications, including end-stage liver disease, recurrent line infections, and loss of venous access. Nowadays with good multidisciplinary IF care, these complications can mostly be mitigated, although with time vascular thromboses and loss of venous access can be critical indicators of failure of therapy. ITx thus is the salvage procedure for those having terminal complications of PN usage. In HD patient who have ultra SGS and are permanently PN dependent, they clearly have irreversible IF and will never come off total PN; however, the consideration and timing of ITx is patient specific and program specific and outside the scope of this review.

INTESTINAL TRANSPLANTATION FOR HIRSCHSPRUNG'S DISEASE

ITx has been performed routinely since 1989, with some cases earlier having been done with poor short-term results. The use of tacrolimus revolutionized the field with better immunosuppressive therapy. Over the last 35 years, ITx has become the established and ultimate therapy for IF. ITx for HD has often been categorized as a transplant for a motility disorder (aganglionosis leading to dysmotile bowel), but essentially it is primarily done for cases of TAG and NTAG which have resulted in SGS. The type of transplant depends on both the patient's needs and the transplant center's practice. The types of ITxs include isolated small bowel, small bowel, and colon, or in cases of liver dysfunction, a liver-containing allograft such as a liver/bowel or multivisceral transplant, with or without the colon. Use of the colon allograft has fluctuated over the years due to perceived immunologic and infectious complications, but nowadays it is routinely used, especially where there is limited or no native colon. At the end of an intestine containing transplant, the "standard" approach in HD (where no attempt or even thought to restore intestinal continuity via a lower connection) has been to form an end ileostomy or end colostomy, although a loop ileostomy and end colostomy approach has also been done. One of the important reasons for a stoma in ITx cases is to gain access to the transplanted bowel for surveillance allograft biopsies to assess for acute cellular rejection (ACR). With recipients who are in intestinal continuity, the stoma can eventually be closed once the early high rate of ACR has lessened. However, in patients with HD, the way to reestablish continuity is with some form of pull-through or J pouch/ileoanal procedure. The concern then is bringing transplanted bowel down to the anorectum with a very low anastomosis. Complications of these procedures in the general (non-transplant) population are already significant; hence, the added fear with using transplanted bowel. A potential concern is related to acute inflammation and reperfusion injury of the intestinal allograft post-transplant that may affect surgical healing of the anastomosis if done at the initial surgery. As well, the recipient is on immunosuppressive agents that may also affect healing. Another key concern is the development of rejection of the allograft, both acute and chronic, that could be severe and cause anastomotic issues, or even require allograft enterectomy. Hence, is it placing the recipient at an undue risk to reestablish connection, so that the stoma can be taken down?

CONTINUITY PROCEDURES AND CONSIDERATIONS IN INTESTINAL TRANSPLANTATION RECIPIENTS WITH HIRSCHSPRUNG'S DISEASE

As mentioned previously, there are several modifications of the pull-through procedure, including the Duhamel, Soave, Swenson, Martin, Ileoanal, and J-pouch style procedures. Each has its pros and cons and is often operator dependent as to which one is employed. The timing of the pull through is also debatable, whether to do it at the time of transplant, or as a delayed procedure when ideally major complications are less frequent. In that way, the recipient would still likely require a stoma initially but can be taken down once the anastomosis is healed after a reconnection procedure.

IS A STOMA REQUIRED FOR INTESTINAL TRANSPLANTATION OR NOT

A question in the ITx field is whether a stoma is needed at all. Recently in non-HD ITx recipients, some centers advocate for no stoma's utilization at all post-ITx and can manage the patient and allograft without it. Clearly if there is not continuity with the lower GI tract, some form of stoma is needed, and this has historically been the case with recipients for HD where there has been concern for performing a pull-through procedure. However, as reviewed in the articles to follow, there are data to suggest that a pull-through procedure can be done in recipients for HD. The transplant team must decide on the relative risks and indication for each recipient and the needs for the stoma, whether for monitoring of ACR or as a diversion to "protect" the lower anastomosis whilst healing. The philosophic, but very real question is whether intestinal continuity is feasible or even advisable, and this then determines the need for a permanent stoma. If a pull through is performed, the stomal question becomes how long does the stoma need to be in place, or if it is even need at all.

QUALITY OF LIFE ISSUES

Of a more general discussion is the quality of life with or without a stoma, whether in a transplanted or non-transplanted patient. There are some patients and families who would do anything to avoid a long-term stoma, whereas others are accepting and understanding and do not want to incur additional possible complications. This discussion is perhaps more philosophic and certainly patient centric although one would assume if the stoma can be taken down it would in most cases lead to better quality of life. The complex question then becomes when to try establishing continuity and whether to perform a diverting stoma that can be used for gaining access for obtaining biopsies. An endoscopic procedure is needed to get the biopsy of intestinal transplant, and through a stoma this is much easier than a transanal approach.

REVIEW OF ARTICLES

There is not an abundance of literature regarding ITx pull-through procedures for HD or similar conditions where a pull-through or ileoanal procedure was performed. Following are some of the most relevant articles on the topic.

In an early article on ITx for TAG/NTAG and intestinal pseudo-obstruction,[1] the investigators comment it is the ultimate therapy for patients with dysmotility syndrome who have end-stage complications of their IF treatment. Although HD is considered a dysmotility syndrome, in the cases requiring intestinal transplant they are really SGS.

Results of ITx in this group of patients are not dissimilar to those found in other ITx recipients, hence no contraindication to transplant. However, they comment on concern with a distal reconnection and functional outcomes in the dysmotile patients This is more related to patients with pseudo-obstruction where an anastomosis has been made to a short segment of preserved distal dysmotile bowel.

In another article "A Meta-Analysis of Clinical Outcomes of Intestinal Transplantation in Patients with Total Intestinal Aganglionosis"[2] the investigators likewise considered ITx a feasible treatment option for patients with very short segment HD. They found 63 patients who had undergone ITx, and intestinal transplant was performed in 37%, and liver-containing intestinal transplant in 63%. The overall survival was 66%. Follow-up was up to 12.8 years post-ITx. Being a meta-analysis from 2003 to 2016, it spans a broad period where management of the liver-related PN injuries were not as well managed as nowadays.

In an article on need for stoma with intestinal transplant recipients "Stoma or no Stoma: First Report of Intestinal Transplantation Without Stoma,"[3] it is debatable but there certainly is literature to suggest it may not be needed after ITx. They claim no stoma to be "an acceptable practice model without obvious adverse impact on outcome." Although this may be true in the non-HD ITx patients, there is no specific comment on patients with HD where ileoanal or pull-through procedures are performed where the indication for the stoma is not just be for protocol surveillance biopsies.

In a more general article analyzing of the use of stomas in ITx "Ileostomy After Intestinal Transplantation: The First in Depth Report on Techniques, Complication and Outcomes,"[4] the investigators found that "most recipients can undergo successful ileostomy formation/takedown." Their analysis of stomas in ITx recipients was that it definitely has its benefits, most can be closed, and complications do not affect survival. Hence, the implication is that after a successful transplant the stomas can in most cases be taken down.

Looking more specifically at articles on pull-through procedures in HD, one of the earliest reports is "Endorectal Pull-Through of Transplanted Colon as part of Intestinal Transplantation."[5] It was a very early initial article (1995) on using pull-through of the transplanted colon using the Soave technique. The 2 pediatric cases were a patient with multiple juvenile polyps throughout GI tract and another with HD. Although the postoperative course was "stormy," which they believed was more related to the complexities of ITx in those early days, both patients were doing well on short-term follow-up. In these cases, the covering ileostomy was closed at 4 months and 1 year with no complications. They believed "this showed the feasibility of the pull-through procedure with transplanted bowel."

In another early article (2003) this time from the French group "Improved Quality of Life by Combined Transplantation in Hd with a Very Long Aganglionic Segment,"[6] the early French experience (1997–2000) outlined 3 patients with liver, intestine, and right colon transplants. The procedure performed was a Duhamel procedure[2] and a Swenson procedure.[1] They were performed 6 to 24 months after transplant. The ileostomies were closed with good functional results 6 to 9 months afterward.

A follow-up paper "Intestinal Transplantation for Total Intestinal Aganglionosis: A Series of 12 Consecutive Children"[7] outlined an updated French series of 12 patients who underwent ITx for HD from 1997 to 2005. Types of transplants included 4 isolated ITx with R colon and 8 liver ITx with the right colon, all with diverting ileostomies proximal to the colostomy. There were 4 deaths/graft failures prior to a pull-through procedure. The pull-through procedures were Swenson[5] and Duhamel.[3] Ileostomy closure prior to pull through were performed in 7. One had sepsis after pull-through requiring a second ileostomy. The subsequent case had the ileostomy reversed after pull-through. Of the 8 pull-through procedures, all were continent, and only one with occasional nocturnal fecal incontinence.

A further article "The Challenges of Closing an Ileostomy in Patients with Total Intestinal Aganglionosis After Small Bowel Transplant"[8,9] mentions that an ITx with end ileostomy (thought to be permanent) was performed on a patient with long segment HD. However, subsequent discussions by the family based on quality of life were held regarding a continuity procedure. They performed a Duhamel with loop ileostomy. There were some surgical intraoperative technical issues related to the foreshortened root of the allograft mesentery, which required some vascular arcade division. The loop ileostomy was closed 2 months later. Subsequently, the patient reportedly was doing well with no complications and having 3 bowel movements a day with normal continence.

In an article "Ten-Year Experience with Bowel Transplantation at Seoul St. Mary's Hospital,"[10] they discussed concern when performing simultaneous pull through at the time of initial transplantation due to theoretic concern for higher incidence of anastomotic failure and prolong surgical time. They recommend making double stomas for a coloanal or ileoanal pull through which was done at 6 to 12 months. Ileostomy closure was performed 6 months later, although they comment this may be delayed in young children for scoping ease rather than having to perform a colonoscopy.

In a related article on pull through procedure, this time for pseudo-obstruction and not HD "Preservation of Native Sigmoid Colon for Secondary Continent Cystostomy After Multivisceral Transplantation for Intestinal Pseudo-Obstruction,"[10] they describe a patient with multivisceral transplantation who underwent a Duhamel pull through using transplanted allograft and loop ileostomy and tube continent cystostomy (Monti procedure) of the native sigmoid colon to manage persistent urinary disease at 15 months of age. The allograft ileostomy was closed 3 months later with good functional results. Although not an HD patient, it goes to show that a pull-through procedure with allograft can be safely performed with good functional results.

In a final article "An Innovative Sphincter Preserving Pull-Through Technique with En Bloc Colon and Small Bowel Transplantation,"[11] the investigators discuss a complicated adult patient with extensive Crohn's disease and ultra SGS. The patient received an intestine colon Tx. A pull through procedure was performed 2 days later. The patient developed ACR on 2 occasions after Tx (day 12 and 78) that was managed with steroids and thymoglobulin. The loop ileostomy was closed 15 months posttransplant. By report, the patient had an excellent outcome, anal continence, and no Crohn's recurrence. This goes to show that even with early ACR, the patient was able to be treated for the ACR and had a good outcome and with no apparent surgical complications.

SUMMARY

HD presents a challenge to restore intestinal continuity in the non-transplant patient, let alone when deciding whether to perform it in a transplant patient. The transplant patient still is at ongoing risks postop, as do the non-transplant HD patients, due to technical issues related to sphincter function and other issues related to the pull through or ileoanal procedure. One does wonder if the ITx recipient may not be subject to some of the postop complications seen in the non-transplant patients such as enterocolitis and other bowel dysfunction as the majority of the supposedly normal "unaffected" ganglionated bowel is not present. This is not to say that ITx is without its own specific set of risks and complications, especially related to rejection and the side effects of immunosuppression. In this discussion, however, the decision has already been made to undergo ITx due to life-threatening complications from PN therapy, so these patients will be living with a transplant anyway. The conundrum is whether intestinal continuity can be safely performed using intestinal allograft, and if so, a stoma is not required in the long run. If not, a permanent-end stoma would remain.

A review of the available literature regarding ITx for HD, stoma utilization, and pull-through procedures utilizing intestinal allograft suggests that intestinal continuity can be safely performed in the ITx patient. Pull-through or other connection procedures can be done with good functional outcome. The timing of the pull through needs to be tailored to the patient and situation. A "covering stoma" will be protective and also allows for assessment of the mucosa but is not essential long term. Like all other ITx recipients, short-term and long-term issues related to the graft need to be managed as with any other ITx case, and although technically challenging, the pull through could be diverted proximally or even taken down and removed if needed.

Very careful consideration and detailed discussion of the risks and complications needs to occur between the transplant team and the recipient needs to make sure it seems to be the correct decision for that patient. Historically, end allograft stomas have been utilized, and this would still be a reasonable "conservative" decision. However, there always is a risk of disuse colitis in the remnant Hirschsprung's-affected rectum. We have recently had a patient who had an ITx many years ago for HD that did not have a pull-through procedure, had recurrent episodes of disuse colitis which the patient was resistant to treat, eventually presented with rectal bleeding and pelvic abscesses likely due to complications of the disuse colitis of this remnant native rectum. Hence, it could be claimed that not doing a pull through may also have its own issues unless the remnant distal bowel is resected very low. Given all the aforementioned discussions and reviewing available data, and particularly considering quality of life issues, establishing intestinal continuity is certainly possible, and with this, a stoma is not required for life.

After a vigorous and interesting debate at CIRTA, the overwhelming vote was that stomas are not required for life.

CLINICS CARE POINTS

- Pull through procedures are standard for most patients with HD, but not without short and long or life term complications.

- PN is a life saving therapy for those with intestinal failure, but have specific complications that can be life threatening.

- Intestinal Transplantation developed as a therapy to salvage those patients having life threatening comlications with PN.

- Intestinal Transplantation is one of the most challenging and difficult transplant to maintain, due to the high immunogenic load and balance of drug therapy to avoid rejection and complications of over immunosuppression.

- Bowel that does not have enteric effluent coursing over it is prone to complications such as disuse colitis.

- Diverting stomas used to protect anastomoses can routinely be closed once the risks of the anastomosis have subsided.

DISCLOSURE

The author has nothing to disclose.

REFERENCES

1. Bond GJ, Reyes JD. Intestinal transplantation for total/near-total aganglionosis and intestinal pseudo-obstruction. Semin Pediatr Surg 2004;13(4):286–92.
2. Nakamura H, Henderson D, Puri P. A meta-analysis of clinical outcome of intestinal transplantation in patients with total intestinal aganglionosis. Pediatr Surg Int 2017;33(8):837–41.
3. Moon JI, Zhang H, Waldron L, et al. "Stoma or no stoma": First report of intestinal transplantation without stoma. Am J Transplant 2020;20(12):3550–7.
4. Dumronggittigule W, Venick RS, Dubray BJ Jr, et al. Ileostomy after intestinal transplantation: the first in depth report on techniques, complications, and outcomes. Transplantation 2020;104(3):652–8.
5. Tzakis AG, Nour B, Reyes J, et al. Endorectal pull-through of transplanted colon as part of intestinal transplantation. Surgery 1995;117(4):451–3.
6. Yann R, Yves A, Dominique J, et al. Improved quality of life by combined transplantation in Hirschsprung's disease with a very long aganglionic segment. J Pediatr Surg 2003;38(3):422–4.
7. Sauvat F, Grimaldi C, Lacaille F, et al. Intestinal transplantation for total intestinal aganglionosis: a series of 12 consecutive children. J Pediatr Surg 2008;43(10): 1833–8.
8. Jazi FS, Sinclair TJ, Thorson CM, et al. The challenges of closing an ileostomy in patients with total intestinal aganglionosis after small bowel transplant. Pediatr Surg Int 2018;34(1):113–6.
9. Grosman J, Aigrain Y, Goulet O, et al. Preservation of native sigmoid colon for secondary continent cystostomy after multivisceral transplantation for chronic intestinal pseudo-obstruction. Pediatr Transplant 2022;26(2):e14180.
10. Chang HK, Kim SY, Kim JI, et al. Ten-year experience with bowel transplantation at Seoul St. Mary's Hospital. Transplant Proc 2016;48(2):473–8.
11. Eid KR, Costa G, Bond GJ, et al. An innovative sphincter preserving pull-through technique with en bloc colon and small bowel transplantation. Am J Transplant 2010;10(8):1940–6.

Should a Stoma Be Used After Intestinal Transplant

Akin Tekin, MD[a],*, Gennaro Selvaggi, MD[b], Brent J. Pfeiffer, MD[c],
Jennifer Garcia, MD[c], Vighnesh Vetrivel Venkatasamy, MD[b],
Rafael Miyashiro Nunes dos Santos, MD[a],
Rodrigo M. Vianna, MD[b]

KEYWORDS

- Intestinal transplantation (ITx) • Allograft (intestine) rejection • Ostomy
- Graft (intestine) monitoring

KEY POINTS

- Graft and patient survival of intestinal transplantation has been improved over the last decade partially secondary to better understanding of allograft rejection and monitoring.
- Standard practice of ostomy creation historically has its own pros and cons.
- Experienced high-volume centers challenged the idea of ostomy formation for every transplant because of potential complications of the ostomies and benefits of not having one.
- Even if the routine use of transplant ostomies is common practice, there are situations where no-ostomy practice can give same graft and patient survival outcomes and avoid complications related to ostomies.

INTRODUCTION

Intestinal transplantation (ITx) is a lifesaving procedure for patients suffering from irreversible intestinal failure and complications from total parenteral nutrition. Over the last 20 years, intestinal and multivisceral transplantation graft and patient survival have steadily improved.[1] This has mainly been achieved at high-volume centers for various reasons (9,10). Despite outcome improvements, the overall number of intestinal transplants is declining due to intestinal rehabilitation advancements and limited availability of transplant centers with the necessary expertise (**Figs. 1** and **2**).[2] Five-year graft and patient survival is approximately 50% and 60%, respectively, from recent scientific

[a] UMMG Department of Surgery, Miller School of Medicine, Medical Campus, University of Miami, Highland Professional Building Miami, 1801 Northwest 9th Avenue, Suite#327, Miami, FL 33136, USA; [b] DeWitt Daughtry Family Department of Surgery, University of Miami, Highland Professional Building Miami, 1801 Northwest 9th Avenue, Suite#327, Miami, FL 33136, USA; [c] UMMG Department of Pediatrics, Miller School of Medicine, Medical Campus, University of Miami, Highland Professional Building Miami, 1801 Northwest 9th Avenue, Suite#327, Miami, FL 33136, USA
* Corresponding author. Highland Professional Building Miami, 1801 Northwest 9th Avenue, Suite#327, Miami, FL 33136.
E-mail address: ATEKIN@MED.MIAMI.EDU

Gastroenterol Clin N Am 53 (2024) 299–308
https://doi.org/10.1016/j.gtc.2024.03.001
0889-8553/24/© 2024 Elsevier Inc. All rights reserved.

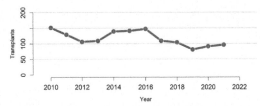

Fig. 1. Overall intestine transplants. Scientific Registry of Transplant Recipients. OPTN/SRTR 2021 Annual Data Report: Intestine. https://srtr.transplant.hrsa.gov/annual_reports/2021/Intestine.aspx#fig:INtx-adult-GF-all-C-inli. Accessed 01-03-2024.

registry of transplant recipients (SRTR) data (**Figs. 3** and **4**). High-volume centers achieved better outcomes with 10-year patient survival of 75% (59% graft) from the University of Pittsburg[3] and 5-year patient survival of 72% by Vianna and colleagues.[4] These improved outcomes may be from better surgical techniques, advancements in immunosuppressive use, greater infection surveillance or control, and cumulative experience in post-transplant management.

Acute cellular rejection (ACR) remains the most serious complication following intestinal transplantation, which directly affects the outcomes along with post-transplant infections. Historically reported ACR rates are up to 40%.[5] Despite common ACR symptoms such as increased stool output, fever, and abdominal pain, some patients may present without symptoms during rejection episodes. This adds greater challenges in determining early rejection episodes and has led to the practice of ostomy creation as a means for allograft surveillance using biopsies and histopathology to determine ACR. Searching for an alternative method for biopsy to diagnose rejection in intestinal grafts has been challenging. Over the last 15 to 20 years, there have been significant searches for potential biomarkers such as granzyme B, perforin, citrulline, and calprotectin.[6] In recent years, studies show a link between high donor specific antibodies (DSA) levels and graft survival, but clinically DSA levels are more likely to predict longer term allograft function rather than early detection of acute rejection.[6–8] Unfortunately, biomarkers have not replaced the gold standard of biopsy even if they can be used as monitoring tools occasionally. In the past, zoom video-endoscopy had been used to support biopsy findings, but its role as to exclude biopsies for rejection was insufficient.[9,10] As a result, we can say that the gold standard for ACR is biopsy and histopathology mainly using ostomies in early post-operative period.

DISCUSSION

Temporary ileostomies are formed routinely in isolated intestine, multivisceral, or modified multivisceral transplants since the established method for intestinal allograft

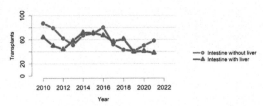

Fig. 2. Total intestine transplants by transplant type. All intestine transplant recipients, including adult and pediatric, retransplant, and multiorgan recipients. Scientific Registry of Transplant Recipients. OPTN/SRTR 2021 Annual Data Report: Intestine. https://srtr.transplant.hrsa.gov/annual_reports/2021/Intestine.aspx#fig:INtx-adult-GF-all-C-inli. Accessed 01-03-2024.

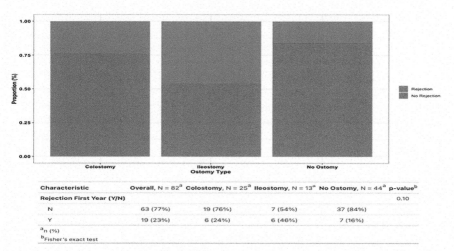

Characteristic	Overall, N = 82[a]	Colostomy, N = 25[a]	Ileostomy, N = 13[a]	No Ostomy, N = 44[a]	p-value[b]
Rejection First Year (Y/N)					0.10
N	63 (77%)	19 (76%)	7 (54%)	37 (84%)	
Y	19 (23%)	6 (24%)	6 (46%)	7 (16%)	
[a]n (%)					
[b]Fisher's exact test					

Fig. 3. Mosaic proportion plot of rejection with 1 year after transplant.

monitoring are regular protocol-driven endoscopies and biopsies. Many centers have different protocols for graft surveillance regarding frequencies, biopsy sides, and clinical symptoms. There are 4 major general types of ostomies used: end ostomy and loop ostomy, and distal and proximal blowhole ostomies. Because every patient has unique complexities, many different adjustments must be made at the time of intestinal transplantation in terms of ostomy formation. Previous surgeries and disease etiology, especially with motility disorders in pediatric patients, may guide which ostomy type should be used. Reported complication rates are very high with ostomy formation 17% to 46% and takedown 13% to 33% procedures, even in nontransplant patients.[11–13] Many different complications are reported including parastomal hernia, prolapse, ischemia, necrosis, volvulus, small bowel obstruction, leaks, sepsis, and fistulas in both formation and takedown procedures. The first detailed report about

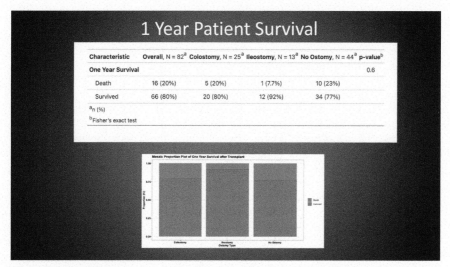

Fig. 4. Mosaic proportion plot of 1-year survival after transplant.

ileostomy-related complications in intestinal transplantation published by University fo California Los Angeles (UCLA) group showed that complication rates were on the higher end of commonly reported outcomes in the nontransplant patient population.[14] They studied patients between 1991 and 2016, including 135 ostomy formation and 79 ostomy takedown procedures. Complication rates were 23.3% and 28% in ostomy formation and takedown, respectively. Almost 70% of the patients in the takedown group required corrective surgical intervention. During ostomy formation, colon-including grafts and high-body mass index patients had greater complication rates. In the ostomy takedown patients, surgical approach was investigated in terms of localized versus laparotomies. Overall takedown complications significantly impacted length of stay. Localized versus laparotomy takedown procedures had similar compli-cation rates but outcomes like operative time, blood loss, and length of stay were favorable in localized ostomy takedown procedures. In this very detailed study, overall complications in both ostomy formation and takedown procedures did not affect the patient and graft survival. This may be explained by greater expertise of the team recognizing and correcting the problems in a timely manner.

Because of potential major complications during the ostomy procedures in intestinal transplantation, the authors' group in Miami decided to take an alternative approach and presented 15 multivisceral or modified multivisceral patient results without an os-tomy in 2015.[15,16] The overall 1-year survival rate was 87% with 2 severe graft rejec-tions and 1 graft loss. This report prompted a question for the necessity of ostomies in intestinal transplantation especially in some high-volume centers. Moon *and col-leagues* from Mount Sinai investigated their routine protocol-driven biopsies and compared them to the study group in which biopsies were only performed if there were relevant clinical symptoms and signs for graft dysfunction such as changes in amount of stoma output and/or characteristics, fever of unknown origin, systemic in-flammatory symptoms.[17] As a result, even with small number of cases, they suggested protocol-driven, routine surveillance endoscopic biopsies do not provide better or earlier diagnosis of acute rejection after intestinal transplantation than clinically indi-cated biopsies. Additionally, they concluded surveillance biopsies in the absence of clinical symptoms and signs did not correlate with higher graft salvage rates from acute rejection. Finally, in the same study, they mentioned that endoscopic biopsies "for cause" only without routine surveillance seems to be effective and adequate to monitor intestinal allografts and was not associated with a statistically greater risk of graft loss or death.

The same group from Mount Sinai published the first report of intestinal transplan-tation without stoma after they abandoned the protocol-driven surveillance endo-scopic biopsies.[18] They compared "Control group" (with stoma), n = 18 grafts in 16 patients and "Study group" (without stoma), n = 16 grafts in 15 patients. One-year pa-tient survival was 89% and 88% in control group and study groups, respectively. One-year graft survival was 78% and 63% in the control and study groups, respectively ($P = 0.378$). There was no difference between patient and graft survival. Cumulative incidence and frequencies of endoscopic biopsies were similar in both groups as well as the renal function. Another important finding was stoma-related wound and surgical complications. They were significantly higher in control group (33%) versus study group (11%) without stoma. These findings were supportive of the idea of a "No-ostomy" approach in intestinal transplantation. The authors' group first presented early results of intestinal transplantation without ostomy in 2015 and then recently updated their results and presented their data between 2013 and to 2022. The authors analyzed n = 82 patients, n = 38 with an ostomy and n = 44 without an ostomy. Rejec-tion episodes in 1 year were similar (see **Fig. 3**), and 1-year and 3-year patient and

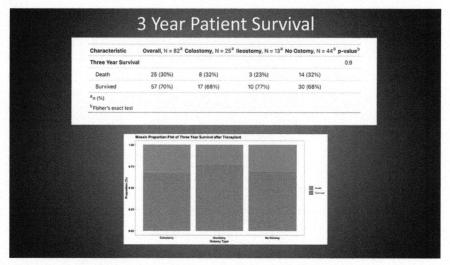

Characteristic	Overall, N = 82[a]	Colostomy, N = 25[a]	Ileostomy, N = 13[a]	No Ostomy, N = 44[a]	p-value[b]
Three Year Survival					0.9
Death	25 (30%)	8 (32%)	3 (23%)	14 (32%)	
Survived	57 (70%)	17 (68%)	10 (77%)	30 (68%)	

[a] n (%)
[b] Fisher's exact test

Fig. 5. Mosaic proportion plot of 3-year survival after transplant.

graft survival showed no significant differences (see **Fig. 4**; **Fig. 5**).They lost only 1 pediatric patient secondary to rejection and no mortality was related to rejection in the adult population. The authors also separately investigated intestinal grafts without liver between 2018 and 2022. Seven out of n = 19 patients did not have ostomy (**Fig. 6**). There were 2 graft losses and 1 patient loss in the "No-ostomy" group, but statistical significance was not reached likely because of very small numbers (**Figs. 7 and 8**).

Characteristic	Overall, N = 19[a]	Colostomy, N = 6[a]	Ileostomy, N = 6[a]	No Ostomy, N = 7[a]	p-value[b]
Gender Assigned at Birth					0.5
F	14 (74%)	5 (83%)	5 (83%)	4 (57%)	
M	5 (26%)	1 (17%)	1 (17%)	3 (43%)	
Ethnicity					0.12
African American	4 (21%)	1 (17%)	2 (33%)	1 (14%)	
Caucasian	8 (42%)	3 (50%)	4 (67%)	1 (14%)	
Hispanic	7 (37%)	2 (33%)	0 (0%)	5 (71%)	
Age (years)	45 (16, 64)	52 (50, 57)	38 (23, 49)	13 (4, 43)	0.2
Weight (kg)	62 (45, 71)	68 (63, 86)	57 (47, 70)	43 (16, 61)	0.047
Donor Gender					0.4
F	11 (58%)	5 (83%)	3 (50%)	3 (43%)	
M	8 (42%)	1 (17%)	3 (50%)	4 (57%)	
Donor Ethnicity					>0.9
African American	2 (11%)	1 (17%)	0 (0%)	1 (14%)	
Caucasian	13 (68%)	4 (67%)	4 (67%)	5 (71%)	
Hispanic	4 (21%)	1 (17%)	2 (33%)	1 (14%)	
Donor Age (years)	12 (4, 27)	16 (13, 23)	14 (6, 26)	3 (2, 27)	0.4

[a] n (%); Median (IQR)
[b] Fisher's exact test; Kruskal-Wallis rank sum test

Fig. 6. Demographics adult + Pedi (n = 19).

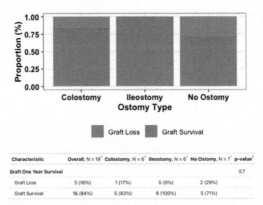

Fig. 7. 1-year graft survival. [1,2], One year survival.

Regardless, intestinal grafts without liver transplantation are at higher risk of loss related to rejection. Therefore, the "No-ostomy" approach should be very carefully considered only in the hands of experienced teams in this group. In both centers practicing the "No-ostomy" approach, patients tended to have better preserved renal function, but the results did not meet criteria for statistical significance. In the authors' group, the authors still individually evaluate cases for the decision of ostomy creation,

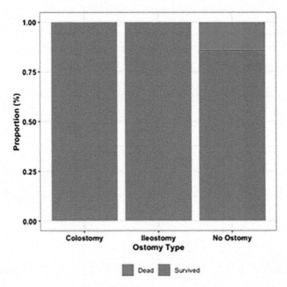

Characteristic	Overall, N = 19[1]	Colostomy, N = 6[1]	Ileostomy, N = 6[1]	No Ostomy, N = 7[1]	p-value[2]
One Year Survival					>0.9
Dead	1 (5.3%)	0 (0%)	0 (0%)	1 (14%)	
Survived	18 (95%)	6 (100%)	6 (100%)	6 (86%)	

Fig. 8. 1-year survival after transplant. [1,2], One year survival.

but they tend to avoid ostomies especially in allografts that include a liver at the time of transplantation.

The discussion here takes few turns when we think in detail. First, we must acknowledge the necessity of histopathology for early diagnosis and treatment of rejection, which is critical for patient and graft survival in intestinal transplantation. Since we do not have reliable noninvasive markers or tools to diagnose ACR, we must rely on our endoscopic biopsies and histopathology. So, the question is whether we can obtain tissue for evaluation through ostomies as we do traditionally or in certain situations, can we use natural orifices and skip ostomies? This "No-ostomy" approach may potentially avoid multiple complications related to ostomy creation and takedown procedures as the authors mentioned earlier. These complications are real, can be life threatening, and costly. Potential benefits of "No-ostomy" approach to avoid all related complications regarding ostomies can be a radical advancement in the field. As shown, the importance of protocol biopsies is in question; the necessity of stoma question is rather problematic. Even though many transplant centers plan to close ostomies in 3 to 6 months after transplant, practically this takes place 6 to 12 months after transplantation.[14] Proximal ostomies tend to produce high outputs increasing the risk of dehydration. This, when coupled with immunosuppression, may contribute to a greater incidence of long-term renal insufficiency in intestinal transplant patients. There is a real possibility of reduced costs related to the potential early discontinuation of parenteral nutrition and avoiding ostomy surgeries and its related complications. There is quality of life benefit for patients, both physically and emotionally, when they do not have to perform ostomy care. Second, we must consider whether this practice is possible in all transplant centers or not, especially when we consider the number of transplants declining over the years and only a few centers reach certain number of cases. So, the experience needed to implement a "No ostomy" approach in general is not feasible in many centers doing only a few cases a year. Even in high-volume and experienced centers, an abundance of caution and discussions need to take place before deciding which patients may benefit and be considered for the "No ostomy" approach. Especially in the pediatric population with motility disorders and the patients who do not have a great amount of native rectal or sigmoid function, it might not be possible to avoid ostomies in the early post-transplant period. Third, there are technical considerations related to availability of abdominal wall and skin for closure. Ostomies might occupy areas which will be needed for difficult closures in terms of skin and fascia availability. Some cases even require abdominal wall transplant because of multiple previous surgeries causing insufficient area to place the allograft and cover with fascia and skin. When this closure issue is a concern, any skin and fascia protective measure might help, so avoiding ostomies may be beneficial. Fourth, patient compliance may dictate the necessity of ostomies. If there are problems with follow-up secondary to various social reasons, an ostomy might be safer by having easier access for endoscopies whenever needed. Another important point to consider in this approach is that detailed pretransplant work up is necessary to determine anatomy and functional status of distal bowel and rectum. This might help to decide whether "No Ostomy" idea can be entertained or not more freely. With healthy and functional distal native colon and rectum, which allows safer anastomosis can decrease the risk of procedure without ostomy.

SUMMARY

Intestinal transplantation (ITx) with or without liver is a lifesaving procedure for patients with intestinal failure and short gut secondary to different etiologies. It is a unique and rare form of transplant in which the graft is highly immunogenic and has the highest rate of rejection compared to other solid organs. The liver-included grafts have a lower rate of rejection potentially due to immunoprotective effect of the liver. Outcomes for both graft and patient survival are slightly better in recent years than before due to many factors including earlier detection and treatment of rejection. Unfortunately, due to the lack of noninvasive biomarkers, the histopathological diagnosis of rejection which requires endoscopic biopsies is the gold standard in early diagnosis and treatment for intestinal graft rejection. To access the graft easily at any time, different types of ostomies have been standard in intestinal transplantation. As the authors mentioned in this article, ostomies come with their own series of complications which can be life threatening. The concept of not having ostomies is relatively recent and not the standard of care. But in experienced centers, it was safely and effectively used with multiple potential benefits, mainly avoiding all ostomy-related complications. Surveillance biopsies are questioned fairly and did not provide early diagnosis and prevention of rejection and did not impact the graft and patient survival in limited studies. So, to have an ostomy for the early diagnosis of rejection purpose only is not justified. Obviously, the number of cases and studies is limited to support "No-ostomy" approach and prospective randomized studies are needed. This can be a challenge, since the total number of cases is not enough and experienced centers who implemented "No-ostomy" approach are only few. Ostomies will still play a vital role in allograft monitoring. Low-volume and less experienced centers should continue to use it as recommended. In a few experienced high-volume centers, the authors will continue to update their results to inform the transplant community to consider the "No-ostomy "approach in suitable cases. When and if "No ostomy" becomes standard, it will be another breakthrough in the field of intestinal transplantation. Whenever we plan intestinal transplant, the pretransplant work up should include distal colon and rectum functionality and patient compliance. Inclusion of liver in the transplant, anatomic concerns, and surgical challenges are also in the equation of this comprehensive evaluation which can guide us to decide whether "No ostomy "approach is suitable for certain cases or not. The authors certainly believe this goal is achievable with detailed planning and gained experience which will help patients' quality of life tremendously by avoiding ostomy-related complications.

CLINICS CARE POINTS

- ACR remains the most serious complication following intestinal transplantation which directly affects the outcomes.[5]

- Routinely monitoring intestinal grafts via ostomies with biopsies has been a standard of care for early diagnosis of acute rejection and treatment for decades[14]

- Ileostomy-related complications in intestinal transplantation are reported 23.3% and 28% in ostomy formation and takedown, respectively. Almost 70% of the patients in the takedown group required corrective surgical intervention[14]

- Similar graft and patient survival rates were reported in a couple of high-volume centers practicing "No-ostomy" approach in intestinal transplantation[15,18]

- The number of cases and studies is limited to support "No-ostomy" approach as standard of care and prospective randomized studies are needed.

- Experienced high-volume centers should continue to update their results to inform the transplant community to consider the "No-ostomy "approach in suitable cases.

DISCLOSURE

The authors have nothing to disclose.

REFERENCES

1. Grant D, Abu-Elmagd K, Mazariegos G, et al. Intestinal Transplant Association. Intestinal transplant registry report: global activity and trends. Am J Transplant 2015;15:210–9.
2. Dumronggittigule W, Venick RS, Dubray BJ Jr, et al. Ileostomy After Intestinal Transplantation: The First in Depth Report on Techniques, Complications, and Outcomes. Transplantation 2020;104(3):652–8.
3. García-Botello SA, García-Armengol J, García-Granero E, et al. A prospective audit of the complications of loop ileostomy construction and takedown. Dig Surg 2004;21:440–6.
4. Fish DR, Mancuso CA, Garcia-Aguilar JE, et al. Readmission after ileostomy creation: retrospective review of a common and significant event. Ann Surg 2017; 265:379–87.
5. Luglio G, Pendlimari R, Holubar SD, et al. Loop ileostomy reversal after colon and rectal surgery: a single institutional 5-year experience in 944 patients. Arch Surg 2011;146:1191–6.
6. Beduschi T, Garcia J, Selvaggi G, et al. Multivisceral transplantation without an ostomy; initial experience with 15 patients, (abstract), ISBTS 2015. In: 14th International Small Bowel Transplant Symposium. Buenos Aires, Argentina, 2015.
7. Moon JI, Zhang H, Waldron L, et al. "Stoma or no stoma": First report of intestinal transplantation without stoma. Am J Transplant 2020 Dec;20(12):3550–7.
8. Horslen Simon P, Wood Nicholas L, Cafarella Matthew. Erin M Schnellinger OPTN/ SRTR 2021Annual Data Report:Intestine. Am J Transplant 2023;23.
9. Abu-Elmagd 1 KM, Kosmach-Park Beverly, Costa Guilherme, et al. Long-term survival, nutritional autonomy, and quality of life after intestinal and multivisceral transplantation. Ann Surg 2012;256(3):494–508.
10. Vianna RM, Mangus Richard S, Joseph Tector A. Current status of small bowel and multivisceral transplantation. Adv Surg 2008;42:129–50.
11. Rumbo Martin, Oltean Mihai. Intestinal Transplant Immunology and Intestinal Graft Rejection: From Basic Mechanisms to Potential Biomarkers. Int J Mol Sci 2023;24:4541.
12. Lauro Augusto, Ignazio R, Marino Cal S, et al. Advances in allograft monitoring after intestinal transplantation. Curr Opin Organ Transplant 2016;21(Issue 2): 165–70.
13. Cheng EY, Wozniak LJ, Venick RS, et al. Clinical impact of donor-specific antibodies on intestinal allograft rejection and survival. Buenos Aires, Argentina: Paper presented at the XIV International Small Bowel Transplant Symposium; 2015.
14. Matsumoto CS, Hawksworth J, Kozlowski S, et al. "Incidence and timing of denovo donor specific antibody in intestinal transplantation. Buenos Aires, Argentina: Paper presented at the XIV International Small Bowel Transplant Symposium; 2015.
15. Kato T, Gaynor JJ, Nishida S, et al. Zoom endoscopic monitoring of small bowel allograft rejection. Surg Endosc 2006;20:773–82.
16. Lauro A, Altimari A, Di Simone M, et al. Acute cellular rejection monitoring after intestinal transplant: utility of serologic markers and zoom videoendoscopy as

support of conventional biopsy and clinical findings. Transplant Proc 2008;40: 1575–6.

17. Moon J, Schiano T, Iyer K. Routine surveillance endoscopy and biopsy after isolated intestinal transplantation-revisiting the gold standard. Clin Transpl 2019;33.

18. Moon JI, Zhang H, Waldron L, et al. "Stoma or no stoma": First report of intestinal transplantation without stoma. Am J Transplant 2020 Dec;20(12):3550–7.

Pediatric Intestinal Failure Associated Eating Disorder

An Overview of the Importance of Oral Feeding in a Population at Risk for Feeding Difficulties

Dana Liza Boctor, MD, FRCPC, MSc[a],*, Tanis R. Fenton, RD, PhD[b],
Olivier Goulet, MD, PhD[c], Cecile Lambe, MD[c]

KEYWORDS

- Pediatric intestinal failure • Feeding difficulty • Feeding disorder • Oral feeds

KEY POINTS

- In pediatric intestinal failure (PIF), oral feeding is important for the development of feeding skills, physiologic adaptation, quality of life and prevention of eating disorders.
- Risk factors for feeding difficulties are common and the impact of their interplay represents a unique paradigm for the feeding challenges encountered in PIF.
- There is a research gap in PIF, but early data suggest that feeding difficulties are prevalent.
- The decision to use enteral tube feeds must carefully weigh the risks and benefits and patient/parental preferences.
- Conventional eating disorder definitions are not applicable to PIF. A PIF-associated eating disorder definition is proposed to include eating skills dysfunction, psychosocial dysfunction, and impact on nutrition support.

INTRODUCTION

In recent years, there has been better survival in pediatric intestinal failure (PIF) and a paradigm shift away from intestinal transplantation due to improved multidisciplinary teams, lipid emulsions, antimicrobial locks.[1–3] Thus, attention has turned to optimizing quality of life (QoL) for those with PIF. There has been long-standing debate on the best

[a] Alberta Children's Hospital, Section of Gastroenterology, Hepatology and Nutrition, University of Calgary, Calgary, 28 Oki Drive NW, Calgary, Alberta T3B-6A8, Canada; [b] Department of Community Health Sciences, Institute of Public Health, Alberta Children's Hospital Research Institute, Cumming School of Medicine, University of Calgary, 3rd Floor, 3280 Hospital Drive NW, Calgary, Alberta T2N 4Z6, Canada; [c] Department of Pediatric Gastroenterology-Hepatology-Nutrition, National Reference Center for Rare Digestive Diseases, Pediatric Intestinal Failure Rehabilitation Center, Hôpital Necker-Enfants Malades, Université Paris Cité, 149 Rue de Sèvres, Paris 75015, France
* Corresponding author.
E-mail address: dana.boctor@ahs.ca

way to feed children with PIF.[4] Most of the literature focuses on parenteral nutrition (PN) and enteral tube feeds (eTF), with very little specifically on oral feeds beyond expert opinion. When feasible, feeding orally is preferred because of the conferred physiologic benefits. Achieving oral feeding skills and healthy eating habits is important developmental pediatric milestones and an important QoL attribute in this population of fragile feeders.[5] The European Society for Pediatric Gastroenterology, Hepatology and Nutrition (ESPGHAN) has recently emphasized that the gastrointestinal (GI) tract should be used following intestinal resection in short bowel syndrome (SBS). Oral feeding is the preferred feeding modality, "as soon and as much as possible" to promote physiologic intestinal adaptation and to avoid feeding disorders.[6] ESPGHAN has recognized oral aversion as an important complication in children with SBS on long-term PN.[7] This review highlights the importance of oral feeding, the risk factors for feeding challenges and disorders in PIF, and what is known about the prevalence of feeding difficulties. Suggestions for how to identify children at risk for feeding difficulties and a proposed definition for pediatric intestinal failure associated eating disorder (IFAED) will be presented.

FEATURES OF NORMAL FEEDING

Learning to feed and eat is a multifaceted process. It has been proposed that the readiness to orally feed be defined as the coordination of sucking, swallow processing, and respiration.[8] The maturation of the feeding process involves a complex interaction between physiologic factors such as cardiac, respiratory, neurohormonal, digestive, sensorimotor, developmental, and parental and infant/child factors.[9] The bidirectional model of feeding considers that the parent has innate characteristics, skills, and resources that interact and respond to a child's innate characteristics, skills, and stage of experimental learning (**Fig. 1**). The responsive parenting style with situational effective strategies leads to food acceptance.[10,11] Positive parental feeding has been described as avoiding food restrictions, allowing children to make their own food choices, and encouraging children to learn self-regulation.[12] In addition to a positive parental feeding style, the other keys to nurturing healthy eating practices include socialization through regular family meals, a healthy home food environment, and associating healthy eating with pleasure (**Fig. 2**).[12] Pleasure in eating has a central role in the development of eating habits in the first 2 years of life and the early social context of feeding may influence food pleasure learning.[13] Nurturing and achieving each of these pillars of healthy eating practices is challenging to achieve in PIF where the context and methods of feeding may be medicalized.

Satter has defined "competent eaters" as those having a positive attitude about food and eating, food acceptance skills that lead to eating an increasing variety of food, skills for internal self-regulation and skills for managing the food context and meal preparation.[14] In PIF, developing competent eaters involves preserving the enjoyment of food while learning to regulate food intake according to symptoms and which foods and amounts may be less tolerated.

DEFINITIONS/TERMINOLOGY FOR FEEDING PROBLEMS

In general, the term "feeding disorder" describes a severe problem resulting in important organic, nutritional, and/or emotional consequences. The term "feeding difficulty" encompasses a variety of feeding challenges and implies that the parent finds it problematic to feed their child.[15] Food fussiness or "picky eating" can be a developmental stage or may reflect mild feeding difficulty. At the more severe end of the feeding difficulty spectrum, nutritional consequences due to feeding developmental delay and/or severe food selectivity raise concern for sensory disturbance or an eating disorder.[15]

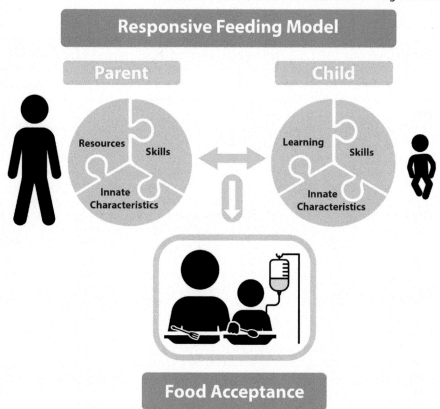

Fig. 1. The parent–child dyad and responsive feeding. Adapted from Ross ES. Flavor and Taste Development in the First Years of Life. Nestle Nutr Inst Workshop Ser. 2017;87:49-58. https://doi.org/10.1159/000448937.

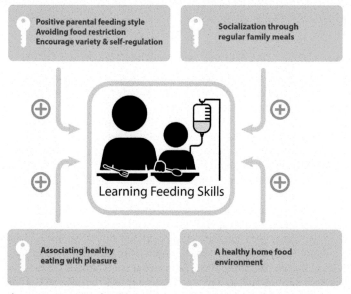

Fig. 2. The keys to nurturing healthy eating practices. Adapted from Haines J, Haycraft E, Lytle L, et al. Nurturing Children's Healthy Eating: Position statement. Appetite. 2019;137:124-133.

Concern is also raised for a feeding disorder if food fussiness persists beyond the toddler developmental phase, and/or if it is creating mealtime discord and nutritional impact.[16] Food selectivity is a feature noted in eating disorders, with children often eating less than 10 to 15 different foods.[17] Each of the features of disordered eating including poor appetite/interest in food, selective intake, and fear of eating[18] may have organic and/or behavioral origins.[15]

The term "oral aversion" relates to the feeding refusal behavior seen in an infant or toddler. This refusal of breast or bottle feeding or complementary foods can be manifest as gagging, vomiting, turning head away from food, or oral defensiveness to sensation in or around the mouth. The definition focus is on the refusal behavior in the young and it does not capture avoidance behaviors in older children or eating skills and psychosocial dysfunction. Thus, the term does not cover the spectrum of feeding difficulty in PIF. On the other hand, the descriptive term "oral sensitivity" relates to the sensory experiences of taste, smell, tactile/texture, and visual stimuli. Oral sensitivity is an important feature of disordered eating, and this can be seen at all ages.

Recently, the expert consensus definition of pediatric feeding disorder (PFD) has been promoted and adopted in pediatrics. This inclusive definition describes an impaired oral intake that is associated with one or more of the following dysfunctions: medical, nutritional, feeding skill, or psychosocial.[19] The nutritional dysfunction criteria include malnutrition or nutrient deficiency or reliance on enteral feeds or oral supplements to sustain nutrition/hydration. This is difficult to apply in the context of PIF where parenteral and enteral nutrition (EN) support aim to compensate for malnutrition or nutrient deficiencies. In general pediatrics, an argument has been made that tube feeding dependency, should be seen as a severe feeding disorder.[9] This is considered with the PFD feeding skills dysfunction criteria (eg, modified equipment or feeding strategies). In PIF, this may also be difficult to apply as the use of eTF may reflect a treatment style/clinician preference rather than a feeding skills dysfunction. The PFD criteria of requiring nutrition support may not be a fair criterion for PIF where the disease drives the need for nutrition support. Furthermore, there may be children with PIF who have healthy eating behaviors.

THE IMPORTANCE OF ORAL FEEDING IN PEDIATRIC INTESTINAL FAILURE
Hyperphagia

In adults with IF, eTF are not commonly used. With decades of feeding skills and food enjoyment preceding the intestinal resection, it is not surprising that adults prefer eating orally after intestinal resection. Those with SBS who are able to manage without PN, compensate by hyperphagia,[20] which has been defined as a food intake exceeding 1.5 to 2.0 times the resting energy expenditure.[20,21] Hyperphagia is prominent in adults with SBS both on and autonomous of PN[22] and is characterized as a behavioral adaptive phenomenon critical for intestinal adaptation and achieving intestinal autonomy.[21] It has been suggested that the most important aspect of dietary management in adult patients with SBS is to encourage hyperphagia.[23] It is unclear why hyperphagia seems to be less common in children. Infants may not have had the hunger and satiety experiences to support the development of hyperphagia if the sentinel event leading to SBS occurs before the establishment of feeds. As well, significant and chronic discomfort from abdominal pain, nausea, or distension in early life may interfere with acquiring skills and learning self-regulation. Contextually, it is difficult to encourage hyperphagia in the neonate and child. The main emphasis needs to be the acquisition of feed skills and learning self-regulation. Excessive pressure from health care providers on parents to "push" feeding may inadvertently negatively impact the parent–child feeding rapport and contribute to feeding difficulties. The consequences of a push for enteral "hyperalimentation" with eTF may interfere with the development of self-regulation. Moreover, overly aggressive eTF advancement may worsen gastrointestinal discomfort and contribute to food avoidance.

PHYSIOLOGIC BENEFITS OF ORAL FEEDING

Epithelial growth factor (EGF) is a trophic hormone known to have an important role in the growth, development, and maturation of the gastrointestinal tract.[24] Data from murine models having undergone sialoadenectomy suggest that salivary-derived EGF has an important role in the adaptive response following massive small bowel resection.[25] The salivary stimulation of this trophic hormone is bypassed with eTF.

The administration of the trophic hormone glucagon-like peptide 2 (GLP-2) analog (teduglutide) has been a major advancement in adult and PIF management.[26,27] In adults, baseline hyperphagia has been identified as an independent predictor for weaning PN in response to teduglutide.[28] In the first pediatric study of teduglutide, 96% of patients on the standard dosing were on eTF according to an algorithm for increasing calories.[27] At 24 weeks, 11% achieved autonomy. In a recent study of 25 children with SBS, one-third of children were completely weaned of PN by 48 weeks. Only 8% of the cohort received eTF at baseline and 12% by the end of the study. The ability to have higher oral intakes was associated with PN weaning, irrespective of small bowel length, citrulline concentration, or absorption rate.[29] Subsequently, it was observed that in 37 children with SBS who received teduglutide, higher oral food intakes were predictive for PN weaning.[30] The intestinal adaptation advantages related to oral feeds highlight the importance of achieving oral skills. At this stage, comparing outcomes with the use of eTF versus oral feeding on GLP-2 is not possible due to study duration differences.

In piglets, the coadministration of GLP-2 and EGF-containing media has been demonstrated to synergistically induce intestinal lengthening and reduce intestinal permeability beyond GLP-2 alone.[31] Although there have not been human trials studying with the coadministration of exogenous EGF and GLP-2; one may speculate that stimulating endogenous EGF by oral feeding, along with teduglutide administration may pose a synergistic opportunity.

The PIF population is known to have a high prevalence of small bowel bacterial overgrowth (SIBO) and this is associated with worse outcomes such as poor growth, prolonged PN dependency, and IF-associated liver disease (IFALD).[32] In healthy children, it is well established that having a varied diet, particularly with different sources of fermentable fibers is important for microbiome diversity. Patients with IF have an overall reduction in the bacterial diversity with more Proteobacteria, Enterobacteriaceae, Lactobacilli, and less Bacteroidetes.[33] The role of whole foods on the microbiome in PIF is not well studied. In a study of 12 children with PIF, the delivery of more than 50% of calories by PN was associated with a reduced bacterial diversity and increased abundance of pathogenic bacteria including proteobacteria and a reduced abundance of Bacteroidetes.[34] This was presumed to be a result of a nutrient-deprived environment for the microbiome and a reduced abundance of short chain fatty acids. Of note, 58% of children were on eTF, 33% received minimal oral feeds, and 67% more significant oral intake. The presence of oral feeds was associated with the abundance of the beneficial Verrucomicrobia and Actinobacteria, a phylum crucial for maintenance of gut homeostasis.[35] Studies evaluating the microbiome in orally fed PIF children in comparison to those on eTF have not been done. However, in children with medical complexity, those on exclusive eTF had less richness in their microbial species compared with healthy controls.[36] It is likely that promoting oral feeds and a variety of complementary feeds would benefit the developing intestinal microbiome in this SIBO prone population.

DEVELOPMENTAL AND PSYCHOSOCIAL BENEFITS OF ORAL FEEDING

Oral feeding is important for the learned enjoyment of food, skills acquisition, and the prevention of feeding disorders.[32,37] There may be a critical window in childhood for solid food introduction.[38,39] The maximal critical window for learning to enjoy new foods is between 4 months and 2 years coinciding with the timeframe when many with PIF are faced with the challenge of learning to eat while being sick and hospitalized and/or on home PN. Achieving feeding milestones may receive less focus because of critical illness, surgeries, and complications of PIF.

A recent study of caregivers highlighted the significant amount of time required for theroutine daily care of children with PIF. In this population, parents reported spending 27% of time on tasks related to eTF.[40] We would expect an improved QoL for the child/caregiver with a reduction in the number of care devices and reduction in the caregiver burden.

Although pediatric QoL studies have not addressed the value of oral feeding, adult studies suggest that the ability to eat food is an important QoL attribute.[41] In a survey of adults with IF, addressing the social and emotional value of eating was identified as one of the key areas for improving QoL.[42] As the parent–child feeding relationship is a fundamental aspect of parental care, we suspect that QoL is negatively impacted in PIF when parents are unable to feed their children normally, whether related to intolerance, nil per os (NPO), strict diets, or the presence of feeding difficulties. Typical pediatric and adult health-related QoL studies do not take into account nutrition or food-related QoL,[43] which has been suggested to be an important adult patient-reported outcome for inflammatory bowel disease and irritable bowel syndrome.[44,45] The SBS-QoL scale[46] includes one item on the influence of disease on eating and drinking habits. Using this tool in adults, oral intake correlated with QoL assessed by the SBS-QoL.[47]

Feeding disorders have a profound impact on the daily lives of children and caregivers.[48,49] In the general pediatric population, literature suggests that the child and caregivers' QoL is severely affected and that parents of children with feeding disorders often suffer from feeding-related anxiety, distress, and attachment insecurity.[9] In the premature infant population, prolonged feeding difficulties increase medical costs, long-term oral feeding aversion, and add to maternal stress.[50] It has been reported that the daily life of caregivers of children with feeding disorders revolves around feeding. Mothering a child with chronic feeding difficulty has implications for social participation, employment status, and future planning.[49] The demands of feeding-related tasks and the resultant feelings of isolation have been described as "living life on the margins."[49]

CONSIDERATIONS FOR FEEDING DECISIONS

Current feeding practice is mostly driven by clinician/center opinion, experience, and preferences. The use of eTF is driven by the hope of decreasing PN dependency more quickly and thus its contribution to IFALD. A study conducted in 15 adults with SBS over a 2-week period observed enhanced nutrient absorption with continuous eTF,[51] which has led some to favor eTF as a strategy to reduce PN requirements. The implication of promoting oral feeds and less reliance on eTF may be an initially higher degree of PN dependence and a slower weaning of PN. For decades, the medical culture in this field has been that PN is "toxic" and needs to be discontinued as soon as possible. However, in this era of less hepatotoxic lipid emulsions and better line care, the risk of IFALD has decreased significantly. A very low prevalence of IFALD was demonstrated in a large cohort where oral feeds were emphasized.[52] Thus, currently, there is less pressure to wean the PN as quickly as possible. Studies that evaluate different feeding approaches with outcomes of morbidity are much needed.

The time to achieve PN autonomy with oral versus eTF has not been studied. Jeppesen has eloquently described that some adults with IF may view PN as a refuge from symptoms and dehydration; others consider PN as a burden and they may be willing to live with hyperphagia and dehydration to avoid a life dominated by a central venous catheter.[53] In a qualitative study of the experiences of PIF family caregiver, poignantly titled "Line care governs our entire world…" families expressed a high degree of fear and stress associated responsibility of central line care.[54] Despite the study of Joly and colleagues[51] demonstrating increased absorption with continuous eTF in adults, eTF are not used as commonly in adults as in pediatrics. In clinical practice, if given the choice between eTF and oral eating, adults with IF prefer to eat. Thus, patient and caregiver preference are an important factor in decisions around oral feeding and eTF.

With eTF, there is a loss of sensitivity to response to a child's hunger/satiety cues and the loss of opportunity for learning self-regulation. In the context of PIF, overfeeding with eTF and resultant increased symptoms is a risk with significant consequences. Concern has been raised that overly aggressive eTF, particularly continuous eTF, in the context of poor motility, and dilated bowel loops, results in increased symptomatology, worsening small intestinal bacterial overgrowth, and resulting in mucosal injury, bacterial translocation, and worsened IFALD.[4] The worsening symptomatology may be experienced as noxious sensory stimulus and thus contribute to eating avoidance or selectivity.

Obviously, there are some situations that necessitate the use of eTF such as developmental limitations in the premature infant or neurodevelopmental delay in the older infant/child and where severe feeding disorders exist that prevent the weaning of PN. As well, in the early postsurgical period of ultra-SBS continuous eTF may be initially required. In this context, several hours off eTF to allow for bacerial clearance is an important consideration.

In considering oral feeding in PIF, it is important to consider that oral feeding has different roles depending on the phase of the journey in PIF and the infant or child's stage of development. In the early premature infant without developmental skills, the goal is to maintain suck and swallow activity whether with nutritive or nonnutritive feeds. In the early post-resection phases of an infant with SBS with high losses or in an infant with pseudo-obstruction with marked symptoms causing significant noxious stimulus; the initial goal is for the infant to learn how to feed. The nutrient contribution at this stage is likely negligible, and the role of feeding is to learn feeding skills. Thus, in the context of significant malabsorption, a small amount orally rather than a couple of cc/hr of continuous eTF would make a significant long-term difference in feeding but only result in a negligible wean of PN in the short term. At the phase of introducing complementary feeds, the goal is for the infant/toddler to learn to enjoy food and the social context. At this stage, providing overly restrictive diet or pressuring the parents with feeding can have long-term consequences. Once adaptation is occurring progressively and significant active PN weaning can occur, the feeds play more of a nutritive role. The intestinal rehabilitation team must relay realistic expectations to parents/caregivers with respect to feed advancement and to encourage patience for PN weaning and an understanding of the need to balance intestinal rehabilitation with the physiologic risks of excessive eTF and the risk of feeding disorders.

FEEDING CHALLENGES IN INFANTS AND CHILDREN WITH PEDIATRIC INTESTINAL FAILURE: A UNIQUE PARADIGM

Indeed, many of the risk factors for feeding difficulties are common in PIF either by virtue of the nature of the disease and/or its treatment. Physiologic and psychosocial factors contribute to the development of feeding difficulties in infants and children (**Table 1**).[15,19] Delayed oral sensory experience and/or negative oral stimuli related to an underlying organic condition may contribute to the features of eating disorders, such as the poor intake/suppressed appetite, sensory/selective issues, or the fear of aversive consequences. The role of chronic GI symptomatology or disease has not been extensively studied; however, a high proportion of patients referred for feeding disorders are reported to have gastrointestinal conditions.[55] In PIF, appetite may also be suppressed by artificial feeding whether PN or eTF. The interplay of risk factors and their impact on the parent–child dyad in the setting of PIF is a unique paradigm as depicted in **Fig. 3**.

PHYSIOLOGIC FACTORS

Many children with PIF may be born prematurely at a time before they have the skills for orally feeding necessitating the use of eTF. Achieving oral feeds in premature neonates has been described as one of the most important, yet challenging milestones[56] with 40% of preterm neonates having difficulty transitioning from gavage to oral feeds.[57] A recent meta-analysis demonstrated that 43% of preterm children experience oromotor eating difficulties between 6 months and 7 years of life and 18% have eating behavior challenges in the early years.[58]

Feeding difficulties in premature infants relate to early physiologic instability, chronic lung disease, and gastroesophageal reflux.[59,60] Those with prolonged ventilation have delayed and altered sensory and oromotor feeding experience during critical developmental periods. With chronic lung disease, there is less effective and less frequent sucking, less endurance, delayed maturation of suck–swallow–breath coordination and the attenuated respiration associated with feeding and related cardiorespiratory compromise can cause distress and prolong the transition to oral feeding.[60] Having an infant NPO is a risk factor based on the obvious delay in feed progression. Higher postmenstrual age at the start of oral feeds was a predictor of feeding difficulties for extremely low gestational age infants and those with feeding difficulties were more likely to have been made NPO for gastrointestinal symptoms before achieving full feeds.[61]

Hospitalized or chronically ill children and especially neonates with the repeated exposure to noxious sensory stimulation with tubes, cannulas and tapes on the face are especially at risk for oral defensiveness and orosensory aversion.[17,60] As well, eTF interfere with the development of oropharyngeal coordination. Children who receive eTF may not get exposed to a variety of tastes and textures in the first year of life.[62] Tube feeding dependency beyond the time when eTF are medically necessary has been associated with oral aversion from negative orosensory experiences, decreased motivation to eat due to a poor perception of hunger and satiety, and limited positive oral experiences.[9,63] Although the literature on oral feeding following eTF is limited, the proposed risk factors for tube feeding dependency and severe feeding disorders include prematurity, chronic medical conditions, and those receiving eTF at 3 to 6 months of age.[9] For those receiving eTF, maintaining sucking

Table 1
Etiologies contributing to feeding difficulties and disorders

Physiologic		
Primary oral sensory-motor skill deficit	Prematurity	
	Developmental delay	
	Structural	
Secondary sensory issue	Delayed oral sensory experience	Prolonged *nil per os*
		Delayed introduction of complementary feeding
		Tube feeds
	Negative oral sensory experience	Intubation/ventilatory support
		Underlying organic condition
		Structural
		Cardiac
		Neurologic
		Metabolic
		Gastrointestinal: esophagitis, gastritis, dysmotility, visceral hyperalgesia
Psychosocial		
Developmental	Language	
	Socialization	
	Cognition	
Mental and behavioral health	Child	
	Parent	
Social	Cultural	
	Loss of family mealtime	
	Parental absence	
Environmental	Chaotic	
	Hospital	

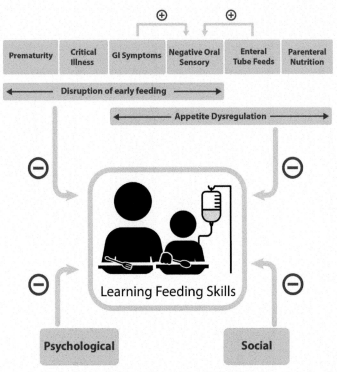

Fig. 3. The paradigm of risk factors for pediatric intestinal failure-associated eating disorder.

with oral stimulation may help accelerates the transition to full oral feeding.[64] Most of the oral feeding guidelines for premature infants now recommend nonnutritive sucking.[59] Children of similar gestational ages may demonstrate variability in the maturation level of their skills.[8] Thus, experts recommend that nutritive and nonnutritive sucking introduction be based on functional maturity rather than gestational age to avoid delays during this crucial developmental period.[60]

There has been very little study on hunger and satiety in the context of PIF. These patients may have a suppressed appetite due to a complex interplay of factors. Lower appetite may be related to disease symptoms and/or the use of EN. It may also be a manifestation of an eating disorder or a "post-traumatic" response where they are afraid to eat[17] due to an experience that has made them orally defensive. Studies in adult are conflicted on whether PN suppresses appetite[22] and there are no pediatric studies in this area.

The timing of complementary feeding and introduction of food texture are important for children with PIF. Even for children without morbidities, delays in food texture introduction beyond 9 months of age are associated with feeding difficulties in childhood.[65,66] In an American survey of 14 centers, the majority had no formal protocol for oral feeding but about two-third consulted occupational or speech therapists to encourage age-appropriate complementary feeding.[67] A working group of the American Society for Parenteral and Enteral Nutrition surveyed dietitian members on their approach to complementary feeding in PIF.[68] Half of the respondents recommended the introduction of complementary feeds between 4 and 6 months, but the vast majority reported that they do not recommend replacing enteral formula with complementary feeds. A survey of 24 European PIF centers observed that only one-third of centers had a feeding protocol and almost all reported a practice of complementary feeding (92%) at 6 months of age.[69] However, in the face of surgical and enteral tolerance delays, beyond the rehabilitation program's stated goals, the actual prevalence and timing of achieving the developmental milestone of complementary feeding milestone is unknown. A recent PIF study reported that purees were introduced at greater than 9 month in 42% of children and that 58% had the introduction of textures delayed to beyond 1 year of age.[70]

PSYCHOSOCIAL FACTORS

Pediatric feeding disorders have a strong relational component.[71] A high conflict parent–child interaction during feeding plays a role in feeding problem development.[19,71,72] Children with dysregulated temperament, mood disorder, anxiety, and/or disordered thinking are at risk of disrupted feeding behaviors.[19] Caregiver stress and/or mental health problems can alter mealtime interactions and how effectively child feeding situations are approached (eg, over- or under-controlling parenting practices).[19,71] Parents may perceive a chronically ill child as more vulnerable and naturally may be more anxious about their nutrition which can lead to pressuring the child to eat which is likely to increase the child's aversive behaviour and decrease intake. A vicious cycle ensues where feeding struggles lead to more vigorous feeding attempts, further disrupting the feeding relationship.[71]

The four fundamental caregiver feeding styles have been described as responsive, controlling, indulgent, and neglectful.[15] The latter three styles can have negative consequences and can contribute to feeding difficulties. Under situations of duress, parenting styles' strengths or weaknesses can be amplified.

The social context of feeding is physically different in the hospital. It is often anecdotally noted that children eat better at home than in hospital. This finding may relate to the child's degree of wellness, the access to quality desirable foods, the inconsistent presence of parents and the effect of acute and chronic duress on parent's feeding skills, resources, and approach. The presence of parents during feeding has been associated with eating behavior and enjoyment of food through both verbal and emotional signals.[13] Infants increased volume of formula ingested in the presence of social interaction.[73] It is difficult for bedside nurses to replace the parental social aspect of feeding during hospitalization. As well, infants and children experiencing medical trauma may have an increased need to exert control over their fractured worlds, which may affect their feeding behaviors. In PIF, prolonged admissions early in life, frequent hospitalizations and clinic visits, chronic symptomatology and disease complexity has become increasingly recognized to have important influences on the development and psychosocial wellness of both children and their parents.[40,74,75]

THE PREVALENCE AND NATURE OF FEEDING DIFFICULTIES IN PEDIATRIC INTESTINAL FAILURE

It is estimated that the prevalence of feeding problems in the pediatric population ranges from 25% to 45% in typically developing children and 33% to 80% in children with developmental delay.[63,76] A recent literature review of the management of feeding difficulties in pediatric SBS identified a major gap in the literature on the prevalence and management of feeding difficulties and feeding disorders.[77] A study of two PIF rehabilitation centers with different approaches to feeding evaluated the frequency of feeding difficulty and disordered eating behaviors.[70] The Canadian center routinely used eTFs and allowed oral feeds as tolerated, whereas the French center promoted oral feeds and aimed to minimize eTF. Using the Montreal Children's Hospital Feeding

Scale[78] to identify feeding difficulties, the overall prevalence of feeding difficulties was 60%. The center that routinely used eTF had higher rates of feeding difficulties, with 39% in the severe range and only 11% having no feeding difficulty. The center that emphasized oral feeding and attempted to minimize any eTFs had 20% in the severe range of feeding difficulty and about half had no feeding difficulty. Although clinicians are concerned that emphasizing oral feeds may increase PN dependence, in this study there was no difference between the centers with respect to the degree of PN dependence. With respect to selectivity as a feature of disordered eating, in the cohort with oral feeding emphasis, 18% ate less than 10 foods versus 41% of the cohort where eTF were used more routinely. The selectivity did not seem to be a function of developmental age. In those subjects greater than 5 years of age, the differences in severe selectivity between the centers were even more pronounced (13% vs 64%).

A national French study of seven pediatric intestinal rehabilitation centers studied the prevalence of feeding disorders defined by the Montreal Children's Hospital Feeding Scale.[79] Among 112 children, the overall prevalence of feeding disorder was 51%, with 15% classified as mild, 8% moderate, and 28% as severe. Several risk factors were studied including gestational age, bowel length, number of surgeries and degree of PN dependence, use of eTF, and bilirubin. The only associated risk factors identified were older age and current speech therapist support. Further research is needed to examine whether those in the severe range may have had associations with the risk factors.

A single center study of 25 patients examined the prevalence of PFD.[80] The practice at this center was to place a gastrostomy post-diagnosis and to use continuous eTF with advancements in volume until feeding autonomy was achieved. Oral feeds were simultaneously provided, and eTF were weaned as skills advanced. Their criteria for PFD were adapted to SBS to include those children that had a reliance on enteral, reliance on high calorie oral supplements, or a reliance on PN. In the first year of life, 100% were considered to have a PFD (with 48% on PN and 85% on eTF). By 4 years of age among the 10 patients that were still followed, 70% had a PFD (20% on PN and 50% on EN). It was acknowledged that eTF support as criteria for PFD was a limitation as the use of eTF may have been an iatrogenic indication given that the use of eTF reflected a treatment style. The study observed that the use of eTF from the time of diagnosis continued to be required well after the patients are weaned from PN. This study prompts the question: if children with PIF have normal feeding behaviors, is it reasonable to consider that they have PFD based on PN or EN dependence?

We studied eating behaviors in PIF using a child eating behavior questionnaire in the study we conducted between the Canadian and French center.[70] Regarding food avoidance, the Canadian cohort scored higher than the healthy UK reference population for food fussiness, satiety responsiveness, slowness in eating, and emotional undereating. In contrast, the French cohort did not differ in the scores other than scoring lower than the healthy UK cohort on emotional undereating. With respect to approaching food positively, the Canadian cohort had significantly less enjoyment of food, whereas the French cohort had the same enjoyment of food as the healthy UK cohort. These differences suggest that normal feeding behaviors are achievable in the PIF population despite encountering many risk factors for feeding difficulty.

The validated Sensory Profile[81] was administered by feeding specialists to in 30 children with PIF.[82] Almost half of the children had high scores for sensitivity to oral touch and taste with 30% scoring greater than 2 standard deviations from the mean. The population scored higher on average for sensitivity to detect sensory input and for avoiding sensory input. These findings help characterize the sensory challenges faced in PIF which will have an impact on feeding difficulty.

Clearly, larger studies and multicenter data are required to gain further insight into feeding practices and the prevalence of feeding difficulties. The International Intestinal Failure Registry included "oral aversion" as the reluctance, avoidance, or fear of eating, drinking, or accepting sensation in or around the mouth.[83] This definition included those who could tolerate partial or full eTF to maintain growth. Those children who could not tolerate eTF due to PIF etiology were not considered to have an oral aversion. In a cohort that has been followed for up to a median of 18 months with age of 1.8 years, the prevalence of oral aversion was 17%. At the 2 month and 2 year follow ups, 67% and 57% respectively were on eTF. This may be an underestimate of the feeding difficulties as the focus was avoidant feeding behaviours and additional features of psychosocial dysfunction such as disruption of social functioning or the caregiver-child relationshiop with feeding and feeding skills dysfunction were not included in the criteria.

FUTURE DIRECTIONS

Treatment is outside the scope of this article and covered the review by Hopkins in this journal. Clearly, treatment is very difficult and behavioral approaches are highly labor- and resource-intensive.[5,9,62] Thus, there needs to be focus on the early prevention of feeding difficulties.

Support to achieve feeding developmental milestones should be included in the clinical care plan of patients with PIF. Infants and children with PIF should be viewed as "fragile feeders" with health care provider cognizance of the individual patient's risk factor profile for feeding difficulty. Patients with multiple risk factors should be identified early for more intensive feeding specialist involvement. There are times when it is not safe to feed, and feeding intolerance may limit feeding efforts. In addition, some risk factors for feeding difficulties such as prematurity and chronic lung disease cannot be avoided. However, whenever possible, concerted effort to minimize the "modifiable" risk factors is important. This would include optimizing opportunities for feeding skills acquisition at developmentally appropriate times and support from feeding and psychosocial specialists. Other opportunities to decrease risks include: minimizing

---

Box 1
Pediatric intestinal failure associated eating disorder (IFAED): a proposed definition

A. A recognition that in pediatric intestinal failure, gastrointestinal symptoms including nausea, vomiting, distension, abdominal pain and/or diarrhea may contribute to the eating difficulties.

B. A persisting disturbance of oral intake with ≥1 of the following:
   1. Feeding/eating dysfunction:
      A. Delay in feeding skills acquisition OR
      B. Eating that is not age-appropriate (texture, quantity, or variety) OR
   2. Psychosocial dysfunction:
      A. Avoidant/selective eating/feeding behaviors OR
      B. Disruption of family relationship and/or social context related to eating OR
   3. Eating difficulties contributing to an inability to wean nutrition support (enteral tube feeding and/or parenteral nutrition) when the clinical situation should allow it.

C. The absence of all the following:
   • Cognitive processes consistent with a body image-distortion eating disorder.
   • Poor oral intake due to food insecurity
   • A diagnosis beyond intestinal failure which is responsible for the feeding problems.
   • A surgical procedure within the last month
   • An acute exacerbation of GI symptoms challenging feeding tolerance

NPO periods when medically safe, and minimizing the use of eTF; in particular continuous eTF, and avoiding overfeeding with eTF.

Specific and brief screening tools for feeding difficulty in PIF have not been developed. Some simple questions that may help identify children at risk include.

1. Does the child have age-appropriate eating? (Consider food texture, variety, and self-feeding)
2. Does the parent find the child difficult to feed? (Consider selectivity or avoidant food behaviors, conflict around feeding and taking longer than 30 minutes to feed)
3. Does the feeding/eating difficulty contribute to the need for enteral or parenteral nutrition support or to the difficulty in weaning nutrition support?

With oral aversion recognized as a possible complication of SBS,[7] an expert consensus definition is required to facilitate identification and introduce consistent terminology for research. Building on the framework of the expert consensus definition of PFD,[19] we propose that a definition of pediatric intestinal failure associated eating disorder (IFAED) should include skills delay, psychosocial dysfunction, or feeding difficulty contributing to the need for nutrition support (**Box 1**). Pediatric IFAED represents a unique and complex set of challenges for the IF rehabilitation team. This problem merits further collaborative research. With the inclusion of oral feeds and IFAED as research variables, we will be able to better understand how to optimize the outcomes in PIF and the QoL of children and their families.

CLINICS CARE POINTS

- Include feeding developmental milestones as part of the clinical care checklist.
- For infants, including those born premature, maintaining suck and swallow opportunities are critical.
- Be cognizant of the risk factors for feeding difficulties, including negative oral sensory experiences such as enteral tube feeds and gastrointestinal symptoms.
- Involve feeding specialist early in high-risk patients.
- Include pediatric intestinal failure associated eating disorder (IFAED) in the problem list of possible complications of PIF.

ACKNOWLEDGEMENTS

We would like to thank Dr Jessalyn Rohs for her contribution of the illustrations used in **Figs. 1–3**.

DISCLOSURES

O. Goulet: consulting for Takeda, Fresenius, and Baxter.

REFERENCES

1. Nader EA, Lambe C, Talbotec C, et al. Outcome of home parenteral nutrition in 251 children over a 14-y period: Report of a single center. Am J Clin Nutr 2016;103(5):1327–36.
2. Goulet O, Finkel Y, Kolaček S, et al. Chapter 5.2.1. Short Bowel Syndrome: Half a Century of Progress. J Pediatr Gastroenterol Nutr 2018;66(Suppl 1):S71–6.
3. Gattini D, Roberts AJ, Wales PW, et al. Trends in Pediatric Intestinal Failure: A Multicenter, Multinational Study. J Pediatr 2021;237:16–23.e4.

4. D'Antiga L, Goulet O. Intestinal failure in children: The European view. J Pediatr Gastroenterol Nutr 2013;56(2):118–26.

5. Hopkins J, Cermak SA, Merritt RJ. Oral Feeding Difficulties in Children With Short Bowel Syndrome: A Narrative Review. Nutr Clin Pract 2018;33(1):99–106.

6. Norsa L, Goulet O, Alberti D, et al. Nutrition and Intestinal Rehabilitation of Children With Short Bowel Syndrome: A Position Paper of the ESPGHAN Committee on Nutrition. Part 1: From Intestinal Resection to Home Discharge. J Pediatr Gastroenterol Nutr 2023;77(2):281–97.

7. Norsa L, Goulet O, Alberti D, et al. Nutrition and Intestinal Rehabilitation of Children With Short Bowel Syndrome: A Position Paper of the ESPGHAN Committee on Nutrition. Part 2: Long-Term Follow-Up on Home Parenteral Nutrition. J Pediatr Gastroenterol Nutr 2023;77(2):298–314.

8. Lau C. Development of suck and swallow mechanisms in infants. Ann Nutr Metab 2015;66:7–14.

9. Krom H, de Winter JP, Kindermann A. Development, prevention, and treatment of feeding tube dependency. Eur J Pediatr 2017;176(6):683–8.

10. Ross ES. Flavor and Taste Development in the First Years of Life. Nestle Nutr Inst Workshop Ser 2017;87:49–58.

11. Satter E. The feeding relationship: problems and interventions. J Pediatr 1990; 117(2 Pt 2):S181–9.

12. Haines J, Haycraft E, Lytle L, et al. Nurturing Children's Healthy Eating: Position statement. Appetite 2019;137:124–33.

13. Nicklaus S. The role of food experiences during early childhood in food pleasure learning. Appetite 2016;104:3–9.

14. Satter E. Eating Competence: Definition and Evidence for the Satter Eating Competence Model. J Nutr Educ Behav 2007;39(5 SUPPL).

15. Kerzner B, Milano K, MacLean WC, et al. A practical approach to classifying and managing feeding difficulties. Pediatrics 2015;135(2):344–53.

16. Fischer E, Silverman A. Behavioral conceptualization, assessment, and treatment of pediatric feeding disorders. Semin Speech Lang 2007;28(3):223–31.

17. Chatoor I. Diagnosis and treatment of feeding disorders in infants, toddlers and young children. Washington, DC: Zero to Three; 2009.

18. Bryant-Waugh R, Markham L, Kreipe RE, et al. Feeding and eating disorders in childhood. Int J Eat Disord 2010;43(2):98–111.

19. Goday PS, Huh SY, Silverman A, et al. Pediatric Feeding Disorder: Consensus Definition and Conceptual Framework. J Pediatr Gastroenterol Nutr 2019;68(1): 124–9.

20. Jeppesen PB, Mortensen PB. Intestinal failure defined by measurements of intestinal energy and wet weight absorption. Gut 2000;46(5):701–6.

21. Crenn P, Morin MC, Joly F, et al. Net digestive absorption and adaptive hyperphagia in adult short bowel patients. Gut 2004;53(9):1279–86.

22. Fourati S, de Dreuille B, Bettolo J, et al. Hyperphagia is prominent in adult patients with short bowel syndrome: a role for the colon? Clin Nutr 2023. https://doi.org/10.1016/j.clnu.2023.09.003.

23. Le Beyec J, Billiauws L, Bado A, et al. Short Bowel Syndrome: A Paradigm for Intestinal Adaptation to Nutrition? Annu Rev Nutr 2020. https://doi.org/10.1146/annurev-nutr-011720.

24. Parvadia JK, Keswani SG, Vaikunth S, et al. Role of VEGF in small bowel adaptation after resection: the adaptive response is angiogenesis dependent. Am J Physiol Gastrointest Liver Physiol 2007;293:591–8.

25. Stern LE, Erwin CR, O'Brien DP, et al. Epidermal growth factor is critical for intestinal adaptation following small bowel resection. Microsc Res Tech 2000;51(2):138–48.

26. Jeppesen PB, Pertkiewicz M, Messing B, et al. Teduglutide reduces need for parenteral support among patients with short bowel syndrome with intestinal failure. Gastroenterology 2012;143(6):1473–81.e3.

27. Kocoshis SA, Merritt RJ, Hill S, et al. Safety and Efficacy of Teduglutide in Pediatric Patients With Intestinal Failure due to Short Bowel Syndrome: A 24-Week, Phase III Study. J Parenter Enteral Nutr 2020;44(4):621–31.

28. Joly F, Seguy D, Nuzzo A, et al. Six-month outcomes of teduglutide treatment in adult patients with short bowel syndrome with chronic intestinal failure: A real-world French observational cohort study. Clin Nutr 2020;39(9):2856–62.

29. Vinit N, Talbotec C, De Tristan MA, et al. Predicting Factors of Protracted Intestinal Failure in Children with Gastroschisis. J Pediatr 2022;243:122–9.e2.

30. de Dreuille B, Mohamed A, Pigneur B, et al. 3: Determinants of parenteral nutrition (PN) weaning in a pediatric cohort of short bowel syndrome (SBS) patients in the era of GLP-2 analogue treatment. Transplantation 2023;107(7S):3.

31. Lim DW, Levesque CL, Vine DF, et al. Synergy of glucagon-like peptide-2 and epidermal growth factor coadministration on intestinal adaptation in neonatal piglets with short bowel syndrome. Am J Physiol Gastrointest Liver Physiol 2017;312:390–404.

32. Goulet O, Nader EA, Pigneur B, et al. Short bowel syndrome as the leading cause of intestinal failure in early life: Some insights into the management. Pediatr Gastroenterol Hepatol Nutr 2019;22(4):303–29.

33. Neelis E, de Koning B, Rings E, et al. The Gut Microbiome in Patients with Intestinal Failure: Current Evidence and Implications for Clinical Practice. JPEN - J Parenter Enter Nutr 2019;43(2):194–205.

34. Talathi S, Wilkinson L, Meloni K, et al. Factors Affecting the Gut Microbiome in Pediatric Intestinal Failure. J Pediatr Gastroenterol Nutr 2023;77(3):426–32.

35. Binda C, Lopetuso LR, Rizzatti G, et al. Actinobacteria: A relevant minority for the maintenance of gut homeostasis. Dig Liver Dis 2018;50(5):421–8.

36. Beauchamp-Walters J, Aleti G, Herrera L, et al. Impact of exclusive enteral nutrition on the gut microbiome of children with medical complexity. J Parenter Enteral Nutr 2023;47(1):77–86.

37. Goulet O, Olieman J, Ksiazyk J, et al. Neonatal short bowel syndrome as a model of intestinal failure: Physiological background for enteral feeding. Clin Nutr 2013;32(2):162–71.

38. Agostoni C, Decsi T, Fewtrell M, et al. Complementary Feeding: A Commentary by the ESPGHAN Committee on Nutrition. J Pediatr Gastroenterol Nutr 2008;46(1):99–110.

39. Fewtrell M, Bronsky J, Campoy C, et al. Complementary feeding: A position paper by the European Society for Paediatric Gastroenterology, Hepatology, and Nutrition (ESPGHAN) committee on nutrition. J Pediatr Gastroenterol Nutr 2017;64(1):119–32.

40. Belza C, Ungar WJ, Avitzur Y, et al. Carrying the Burden: Informal Care Requirements by Caregivers of Children with Intestinal Failure Receiving Home Parenteral Nutrition. J Pediatr 2022;250:75–82.e3.

41. Winkler MF, Wetle T, Smith C, et al. The meaning of food and eating among home parenteral nutrition-dependent adults with intestinal failure: A qualitative inquiry. J Am Diet Assoc 2010;110(11):1676–83.

42. Blüthner E, Bednarsch J, Stockmann M, et al. Determinants of Quality of Life in Patients With Intestinal Failure Receiving Long-Term Parenteral Nutrition Using the SF-36 Questionnaire: A German Single-Center Prospective Observational Study. JPEN - J Parenter Enter Nutr 2020;44(2):291–300.

43. Itani L, Sammarco R, El Ghoch M. Editorial: Nutrition and Health-Related Quality of Life: Is It an Ignored Outcome? Front Nutr 2021;8:778816.

44. Guadagnoli L, Mutlu EA, Doerfler B, et al. Food-related quality of life in patients with inflammatory bowel disease and irritable bowel syndrome. Qual Life Res 2019;28(8):2195–205.

45. Whelan K, Murrells T, Morgan M, et al. Food-related quality of life is impaired in inflammatory bowel disease and associated with reduced intake of key nutrients. Am J Clin Nutr 2021;113(4):832–44.

46. Berghöfer P, Fragkos KC, Baxter JP, et al. Development and validation of the disease-specific Short Bowel Syndrome-Quality of Life (SBS-QoL^{TM}) scale. Clin Nutr 2013;32(5):789–96.

47. Bednarsch J, Blüthner E, Karber M, et al. Oral intake and plasma citrulline predict quality of life in patients with intestinal failure. Nutrition 2020;79–80.

48. Simione M, Dartley AN, Cooper-Vince C, et al. Family-centered Outcomes that Matter Most to Parents: A Pediatric Feeding Disorders Qualitative Study. J Pediatr Gastroenterol Nutr 2020;71(2):270–5.

49. Hewetson R, Singh S. The lived experience of mothers of children with chronic feeding and/or swallowing difficulties. Dysphagia 2009;24(3):322–32.

50. Lau C. Development of infant oral feeding skills: what do we know? Am J Clin Nutr 2016;103(2):616S–21S.

51. Joly F, Dray X, Corcos O, et al. Tube Feeding Improves Intestinal Absorption in Short Bowel Syndrome Patients. Gastroenterology 2009;136(3):824–31.

52. Goulet O, Breton A, Coste ME, et al. Pediatric Home Parenteral Nutrition in France: A six years national survey. Clin Nutr 2021;40(10):5278–87.

53. Jeppesen PB, Fuglsang KA. Nutritional Therapy in Adult Short Bowel Syndrome Patients with Chronic Intestinal Failure. Gastroenterol Clin N Am 2018;47(1): 61–75.

54. Belza C, Patterson C, Ghent E, et al. "Line care governs our entire world": Understanding the experience of caregivers of children with intestinal failure receiving long-term parenteral nutrition. JPEN - J Parenter Enter Nutr 2022;46(7):1602–13.

55. Rivera-Nieves D, Conley A, Nagib K, et al. Gastrointestinal Conditions in Children With Severe Feeding Difficulties. Glob Pediatr Health 2019;6. 2333794X19838536.

56. da Rosa Pereira K, Levy DS, Procianoy RS, et al. Impact of a pre-feeding oral stimulation program on first feed attempt in preterm infants: Double-blind controlled clinical trial. PLoS One 2020;15(9 September).

57. Jadcherla S. Dysphagia in the high-risk infant: potential factors and mechanisms. Am J Clin Nutr 2016;103(2). 622S-8S.

58. Walton K, Daniel AI, Mahood Q, et al. Eating Behaviors, Caregiver Feeding Interactions, and Dietary Patterns of Children Born Preterm: A Systematic Review and Meta-Analysis. Adv Nutr 2022;13(3):875–912.

59. Bakker L, Jackson B, Miles A. Oral-feeding guidelines for preterm neonates in the NICU: a scoping review. J Perinatol 2021;41(1):140–9.

60. Viswanathan S, Jadcherla S. Feeding and Swallowing Difficulties in Neonates: Developmental Physiology and Pathophysiology. Clin Perinatol 2020;47(2): 223–41.

61. Patra K, Greene MM. Impact of feeding difficulties in the NICU on neurodevelopmental outcomes at 8 and 20 months corrected age in extremely low gestational age infants. J Perinatol 2019;39(9):1241–8.

62. Mason SJ, Harris G, Blissett J. Tube feeding in infancy: Implications for the development of normal eating and drinking skills. Dysphagia 2005;20(1):46–61.

63. Bernard-Bonnin AC. Feeding problems of infants and toddlers. Can Fam Physician 2006;52(10):1247–51.

64. Greene Z, O'Donnell CP, Walshe M. Oral stimulation for promoting oral feeding in preterm infants. Cochrane Database Syst Rev 2016;9(9):CD009720.

65. Northstone K, Emmett P, Nethersole F. The effect of age of introduction to lumpy solids on foods eaten and reported feeding difficulties at 6 and 15 months. J Hum Nutr Diet 2001;14(1):43–54.

66. Coulthard H, Harris G, Emmett P. Delayed introduction of lumpy foods to children during the complementary feeding period affects child's food acceptance and feeding at 7 years of age. Matern Child Nutr 2009;5(1):75–85.

67. Nucci AM, Ellsworth K, Michalski A, et al. Survey of Nutrition Management Practices in Centers for Pediatric Intestinal Rehabilitation. Nutr Clin Pract 2018;33(4):528–38.

68. Nucci AM, Samela K, Bobo E, et al. Complementary food introduction practices in infants with intestinal failure. Nutr Clin Pract 2023;38(1):177–86.

69. Verlato G, Hill S, Jonkers-Schuitema C, et al. Results of an International Survey on Feeding Management in Infants With Short Bowel Syndrome-Associated Intestinal Failure. J Pediatr Gastroenterol Nutr 2021;73(5):647–53.

70. Boctor DL, Jutteau WH, Fenton TR, et al. The prevalence of feeding difficulties and potential risk factors in pediatric intestinal failure: Time to consider promoting oral feeds? Clin Nutr 2021;40(10):5399–406.

71. Davies WH, Satter E, Berlin KS, et al. Reconceptualizing feeding and feeding disorders in interpersonal context: The case for a relational disorder. J Fam Psychol 2006;20(3):409–17.

72. Chatoor I. Feeding disorders in infants and toddlers: diagnosis and treatment. Child Adolesc Psychiatr Clin N Am 2002;11(2):163–83.

73. Lumeng JC, Patil N, Blass EM. Social influences on formula intake via suckling in 7 to 14-week-old-infants. Dev Psychobiol 2007;49(4):351–61.

74. Bondi BC, Gold A, Belza C, et al. Predictors of Social-Emotional Development and Adaptive Functioning in School-Age Children with Intestinal Failure. J Clin Psychol Med Settings 2023;30(3):589–605.

75. McCaig JK, Henry OS, Stamm DA, et al. Generic and Disease-specific Health-related Quality of Life in Pediatric Intestinal Failure. J Pediatr Gastroenterol Nutr 2021;73(3):338–44.

76. Linscheid TR, Budd KS, Rasnake LK. Pediatric feeding problems. In: Handbook of pediatric Psychology. 3rd Ed. The Guilford Press; 2003. p. 481–98.

77. Gigola F, Carletti V, Coletta R, et al. Treatment of Food Aversion and Eating Problems in Children with Short Bowel Syndrome: A Systematic Review. Children 2022;9(10). https://doi.org/10.3390/children9101582.

78. Ramsay M, Martel C, Porporino M, et al. The Montreal Children's Hospital Feeding Scale: A Brief Bilingual Screening Tool for Identifying Feeding Problems. Paediatr Child Health 2011;16. https://doi.org/10.1093/pch/16.3.147.

79. Di Mari C, Lambe C, Ecochard-Dugelay E, et al. Feeding disorder in children with intestinal failure on home parenteral nutrition: prevalence and associated factors. ESPGHAN 54th Annual Meeting Abstracts. J Pediatr Gastroenterol Nutr 2022; 74(S2):1144–5.

80. Christian VJ, Van Hoorn M, Walia CLS, et al. Pediatric Feeding Disorder in Children With Short Bowel Syndrome. J Pediatr Gastroenterol Nutr 2021; 72(3):442–5.
81. Dunn W. The sensations of everyday life: empirical, theoretical, and pragmatic considerations. Am J Occup Ther 2001;55(6):608–20.
82. Boctor D, Delacour L, David CB, et al. P3B. 19: The sensory profile of children with Intestinal Failure. Transplantation 2019;103(7S2):S56.
83. Avitzur Y, Pahl E, Venick R. The Development of the International Intestinal Failure Registry and Overview of its Results. Eur J Pediatr Surg 2023. https://doi.org/10.1055/a-2212-6874.

Strategies to Promote Success in Oral Feedings in Infants and Children with Intestinal Failure due to Short Bowel Syndrome

Judy Hopkins, OTD, OT/L, SWC[a],*, Russell Merritt, MD, PhD[b,c]

KEYWORDS

- Oral feeding • Parenteral nutrition • Pediatric feeding disorders
- Short bowel syndrome • Intestinal failure • Avoidant restrictive food intake disorder
- Multidisciplinary care teams • Parent education

KEY POINTS

- Pediatric feeding disorders related to intestinal failure, short bowel syndrome, and other complex medical conditions can impede an infant or child's ability to attain enteral autonomy through oral feeding.
- Feeding problems can present as feeding aversion; difficulty chewing, ingesting, or swallowing food; altered nutritional status caused by insufficient intake, malabsorption, or increased losses; difficulty in the parent/caregiver–child feeding dynamic; or social dysfunction related to the feeding problem.
- There are several practical strategies that a multidisciplinary care team can use to help promote oral feeding in infants and children with pediatric feeding disorder (PFD) or avoidant/restrictive food intake disorder, addressing both motor sensory challenges and psychological and social factors.
- Parent education by the care team is crucial, and children with PFD greatly benefit from parents' dedication to addressing the challenges of oral feeding at home by engaging in responsive feeding and finding ways to include the child at family mealtime.

BACKGROUND

Because feeding is an important aspect of infant and child development, it commonly gives rise to parental concerns and complaints in general pediatric as well as pediatric

[a] Division of Occupational Therapy, Children's Hospital Los Angeles, Los Angeles, CA, USA;
[b] Division of Gastroenterology, Hepatology and Nutrition, Children's Hospital Los Angeles;
[c] Department of Pediatrics, Keck School of Medicine, University of Southern California, Los Angeles, CA, USA
* Corresponding author. 4650 Sunset Boulevard MS #56, Los Angeles, CA 90027.
E-mail address: jhopkins@chla.usc.edu

Gastroenterol Clin N Am 53 (2024) 329–341
https://doi.org/10.1016/j.gtc.2024.01.008
0889-8553/24/© 2024 Elsevier Inc. All rights reserved.
gastro.theclinics.com

gastrointestinal (GI) practices. Up to 50% of parents may express concerns about a child's feeding, whereas the percentage is in the 80% range for those with children with neurodevelopmental disorders.[1-3] Children with a history of prematurity[4] or short bowel syndrome (SBS)—who may also have a history of prematurity—carry increased risk.[4-6] Recently, there have been updates in the diagnostic terms used to describe medically significant feeding problems. These include pediatric feeding disorders (PFDs; the WHO International Disease Classification International Disease Classification [ICD]-10, 2020, R63.31 for acute or R63.32 for chronic) and avoidant/restrictive food intake disorder (ARFID; Diagnostic and Statistical Manual of Mental Health Disorders of the American Psychiatric Association [DSM-V], 2013 and ICD10-F50.82). In this article, the authors focus on oral feeding strategies for infants and children with intestinal failure and related PFD. The authors will not discuss ARFID in detail; milder feeding problems, for example, picky eating; parental misperceptions about feeding and growth; or the eating (vs feeding) disorders more common in adolescents and adults.

PFD is defined as inappropriate oral intake of greater than 2-week duration with medical dysfunction (eg, cardiorespiratory symptoms during feeding or signs of aspiration; nutritional dysfunction, including reliance on enteral feedings or supplements; feeding skill dysfunction requiring alterations in food or the feeding process; and/or psychosocial dysfunction related to difficult feeding behavior).[7] Per the DSM-V, ARFID is a mental health diagnosis that can be made at any age for which patients must have:

An eating or feeding disturbance (eg, apparent lack of interest in eating or food; avoidance based on the sensory characteristics of food; concern about aversive consequences of eating) as manifested by persistent failure to meet appropriate nutritional and/or energy needs associated with one (or more) of the following.

1. Significant weight loss (or failure to achieve expected weight gain or faltering growth in children).
2. Significant nutritional deficiency.
3. Dependence on enteral feeding or oral nutritional supplements.
4. Marked interference with psychosocial functioning.

The findings cannot be due to an underlying medical disorder, cultural practice, or an eating disorder such as anorexia nervosa.

Infants and children presenting with feeding problems may display a lack of interest in eating; fear of feeding; preferences of various degrees for some foods and not others; difficulty ingesting, chewing, and/or swallowing food; failure to gain weight; weight loss and/or nutrient deficiencies; and psychosocial or developmental pathology that may be at least partially etiologic or may be a resultant morbidity. The feeding problem may be grounded in anatomic, physiologic, or medical pathology or can be largely behavioral at the patient or caretaker–child dyad level.

The underlying anatomic, physiologic, and developmental pathology may be exacerbated by responses of caretakers frustrated with the atypical infant response to attempted oral feeding. The parent may give up on oral feedings altogether, force oral feedings, or resort to distracting mealtime behaviors (eg, "Here comes the airplane"). This may sometimes be happening in parents who, themselves, have not experienced sufficient nurturing as children and may be experiencing difficulties adapting to parenthood, or who have been physically separated from their neonate for medical reasons for an extended period. As for the infant, she often learns and displays protective avoidant behaviors that exacerbate parent–child conflict over feeding. Given their complex medical and developmental histories, these children are at increased risk for malnutrition and micronutrient deficiencies not only early on with their intestinal failure but also while, and after, being weaned from previously effective nutritional support.[8]

Intestinal failure is defined broadly as "the reduction of gut function below the minimum necessary for the absorption of macronutrients and/or water and electrolytes, such that intravenous support is required to maintain health and/or growth."[9] Pediatric intestinal failure has been defined more specifically as "the reduction of functional intestinal mass below that which can sustain life, resulting in dependence on supplemental parenteral support for a minimum of 60 days within a 74 consecutive day interval."[10]Pediatric SBS is "the need for PN [parenteral nutrition] for >60 days after intestinal resection or a bowel length of <25% of expected."[11] The vast majority of pediatric patients with SBS experienced congenital or acquired neonatal conditions (most commonly gastroschisis, bowel atresia, malrotation with volvulus, and necrotizing enterocolitis [NEC]) leading to severe medical morbidity before they learn how to eat. The critical goal of treatment for children with SBS is to promote the process of bowel adaptation such that the intestine grows and intestinal function improves sufficiently over time so the child will no longer be dependent on parenteral nutrition (PN).[11] If enteral feeding is used as part of this transition, the goal then becomes weaning from that to oral feeding.

Patients with intestinal failure due to short gut syndrome who have feeding problems present in a manner distinct from other infants and children with feeding problems. They are already receiving gastrointestinal, surgical, and often multidisciplinary care for their intestinal failure. The underlying cause of infant-onset intestinal failure may have made oral feeding impossible or limited for a prolonged time early in life, leading to delay in the start of enteral feeding and adverse experiences associated with feeding attempts (eg, pain, vomiting, distension, aspiration, and diarrhea).[5] Either or both of these mechanisms have long been known to be associated with the development of feeding problems. These children may display both food refusal and highly selective feeding choices. Intestinal failure leads to nutritional deficits (unless avoided by early nutrition support) and family stress associated with the initial hospitalization and subsequently with home nutritional support, including caretaker sleep deprivation, and worry about potential complications of home care.[12,13] Many infants with SBS have comorbidities including prematurity, developmental delay, behavioral issues, and/or parental poverty.[14,15] SBS increases the developmental morbidity associated with prematurity.[16] It is not uncommon for parents of infants who require neonatal intensive care to develop symptoms of post-traumatic stress disorder.[17]

The initial life-saving therapy for these children including surgery, PN, and treatment of their comorbidities may place support of normal feeding development at low priority, whereas in some cases, depending on the underlying gastrointestinal condition and its severity, normal feeding development may be impossible. In addition to receiving PN, many of these children undergo placement of surgical gastrostomies to facilitate upper gastrointestinal drainage or enteral feeding. Those with gastrostomies may be less likely to progress readily with oral feeding.[18]

Given that feeding problems developing in children with SBS are largely grounded in the underlying disease, a diagnosis of PFD will most often be appropriate and has been used for these patients.[6] However, many of the behaviors and nutritional, psychological, and social consequences are consistent with what is seen in patients diagnosed with ARFID and the subtypes associated with this diagnosis.[19,20] In some patients, when the child's bowel has adapted sufficiently, and the child is no longer dependent on PN, the remaining challenges (such as weaning the child from enteral tube feeding to oral feeding) may fit as well with the ARFID paradigm as PFD.

Assessments

Some children with intestinal failure can gain skills and maintain interest in oral feeding despite their medical condition. However, there are "red flags" (**Box 1**) that indicate an

---

Box 1
Red flags for feeding and swallowing disorders

Poor weight gain

Coughing, choking, or gagging

Refusal to eat certain textures

Eats less than 20 foods

Meals take longer than 30 minutes

Difficulty transitioning to food tastes or textures

Negative behaviors during mealtime

---

infant or child may need more support/additional strategies to achieve enteral autonomy through oral feeding.

Altered nutritional status

A major source of morbidity with PFD is altered nutritional status related to insufficient food intake and/or highly selective food intake that can risk micronutrient deficiencies.[21] Insufficient food intake leads to what historically has been termed "failure to thrive," with infants and children falling off weight and height growth percentile charts and is now—perhaps more appropriately—termed weight faltering, growth faltering, or pediatric undernutrition.[22–24] Infants and children are categorized as mildly, moderately, or severely malnourished based on height, weight, and body mass index (BMI) attainment for age. Those affected by feeding problems often have not only a feeding problem-related diagnosis but also a diagnosis of mild, moderate, or severe malnutrition of variable causation.[25,26] Malnutrition may need to be the initial focus of therapy, depending on the severity.[27]

STRATEGIES

Many authors have addressed the feeding challenges for children with intestinal failure, but few provide practical approaches to help support oral feeding. We place the strategies to promote oral feeding into three categories: (1) infancy, (2) childhood, and (3) parent education/support. We present several methods within these categories, explaining the significance of each strategy and offering details about practical application in a clinical setting or by parents and caregivers at home.

Although these practices are offered from a context of occupational therapy, they do not require an occupational therapist to use them. Rather, they can be incorporated into a multidisciplinary care team's approach and, for example, carried out by a psychologist, dietician, or dedicated nurse, as well as taught to caregivers to use at home.

Infancy

Strategy: early introduction of oral feeds

Oral and/or enteral nutrition should be started in a small volume and increased slowly based on tolerance. The first year of life is a critical period for the development of oral feeding skills, and this window of opportunity for learning how to eat orally should be respected and supported. If this period is missed, children may display oral-motor, sensory, and developmental feeding problems when they are weaned off PN and/or enteral tube feeding.[28] Gigola and colleagues provide a good analysis of the relationship between infants with SBS and this crucial period in their oral feeding development:

"Comorbidities associated with SBS, or SBS itself, may determine the delayed introduction of food by mouth in affected children; this could impact later food choices and feeding development. Suppose an infant experiences negative stimuli in the oral cavity in the first phase of life, such as tube insertion, oral hygiene, and suctioning. In that case, the child could correlate oral feeding with stressful experiences, possibly leading to FA [feeding aversion]. In 1964, Illingworth and colleagues postulated the existence of 'critical windows,' specific periods in which children should be offered solid food to develop oral skills. If children are not offered solid food when they learn to chew, they could develop difficulties introducing these foods later on. To avoid FA, oral nutrition should be started as soon as possible with breast milk or formula, and critical windows can be exploited to help the child to develop feeding skills."[5]

If it is possible, oral feeding is preferred to enteral feeding because the former promotes epidermal growth factor release from salivary glands, for bowel adaptation increases GI secretion of trophic factors, and helps prevent feeding disorders.[28] Further, in a 2023 paper, Norsa and colleagues showed that enteral nutrition and establishment of oral feeding play a fundamental role in stimulating bowel adaptation and promoting enteral autonomy.[29]

When oral feeds are not possible or not yet possible, oral stimulation techniques can encourage the development of oral feeding skills during the critical window when the feeding behaviors are reflexive. Oral stimulation during this period facilitates the learning of sucking and swallowing skills and help the infant maintain the learned skills after the reflexive period required for early feeding is over.[30] (See the next strategy for more on oral stimulation.)

Practical application. To practice this in a clinical setting, there are several methods available, which depend on the patient's feeding tolerance. Either of these approaches can be used at a frequency of twice a day when the infant is awake and alert.

- Offer a small volume of breast milk or formula via a bottle.
- If a bottle cannot be tolerated, offer tastes of breast milk or formula using a pacifier, a gloved finger, or a toothette.

Strategy: nonnutritive pre-feeding oral stimulation when oral feeds are not possible
Oral motor intervention and nonnutritive sucking (NNS) can be used for promoting oral feeding skills in preterm infants. Typically, oral stimulation techniques are based on Beckman Oral Motor Intervention that uses a variety of exercises that stimulate the oral structures to improve the strength, coordination, awareness, and range of motion of the tongue, cheeks, lips, and jaw. NNS is stimulated with a gloved finger, pacifier, or nipple without the introduction of food. Strong evidence supports the use of perioral and intraoral stimulation for pre-feeding readiness and preparation to promote successful oral feeding in preterm infants.[31] These approaches provide sensory and motor experiences that have been shown to be effective in facilitating the development of oral feeding skills. Oral motor intervention combined with NNS can also be used to improve the oral motor ability of infants with SBS and possibly reduce the occurrence of adverse effects related to food aversion.[32]

Practical application. One can follow an oral stimulation program proposed by Fucile and colleagues, which prescribes 12 minutes of stroking the cheeks in a circular motion and stroking the vestibular region of the lips, gums, and tongue with the fingertips in an anteroposterior direction, followed by a final 3 minutes of NNS.[33] Occupational therapists can teach parents this technique so they can provide oral stimulation, whereas the infant is hospitalized as well as post-discharge.

Childhood

Strategy: introduction of complementary feeds at developmentally appropriate ages
Introducing solids with a variety of textures and flavors at developmentally appropriate ages facilitates progression of chewing, swallowing, and oral intake. Transition to solid foods is an important stage in development and nutrition. Altered early feeding development may affect food choices throughout childhood. Mennella and Trabulsi found that when infants were introduced to solid foods at age ≥10 months, they ate fewer foods of all types and were less likely to eat table food at 15 months of age.[34]

Another study involving the introduction of lumpy solids suggested that early exposure to varied textures and flavors is important not only for later food choices but also for feeding development.[35] If the child's medical condition does not allow oral feeding during these critical periods, the child may display oral motor, sensory, and developmental feeding problems when attempts are made to start oral feeding at a later age.[30]

An international survey of enteral feeding practices in infants with SBS revealed similarities in the introduction of complementary feedings, but with wide variation in the specific foods introduced relative to textures (eg, lumpy, smooth, or crunchy) and types (eg, vegetables, meat, and other proteins).[36]

Practical application. There are a variety of factors to consider before and during the implementation of this approach, including timing, infant or child readiness, and the foods and techniques used (see **Table 1**).

Strategy: Mealtime participation

An important practice in promoting oral feeding skills in children with intestinal failure is to facilitate their participation as much as possible in family mealtime. For the healthy child, feeding typically occurs at mealtimes, and these experiences happen within a social context wherein a parent reads and responds to a child's feeding cues.[37] By including a child with PFD in family mealtime, the child reaps the benefit of social connection within the family. This strategy also helps the child acclimate to the sight and smell of food, even before oral feeding is possible.

Table 1
What to consider when introducing complementary feeds as a strategy to support oral feeding

Consideration	Description
Timing	The American Academy of Pediatrics recommends introducing complementary foods at approximately 6 months of age.
Readiness signs	Look for signs that the infant is ready for solid foods, such as: • *Sitting up.* The infant should be able to sit up with support. • *Interest in food.* The infant shows interest in watching others eat, or they begin reaching for food.
Foods	Start with single-ingredient, pureed or soft mashed vegetables. As the infant gets used to mashed and pureed foods, you can gradually increase the texture of the food to more lumpy or firmer mashed textures.
Equipment	Use a high chair to support the infant's sitting position during feedings.
Feeding schedule	Start with one meal a day and gradually increase to two or three meals.
Feeding technique	When introducing solids, feed the infant small amounts, about one to two teaspoons at a time. Watch for feeding cues (eg, turning away from the spoon) and stop if the infant is not interested.

Family meals hold more significance than simply a time for nourishment. Fiese and colleagues found that family mealtimes strengthened family identity and offered opportunities for direct communication and problem-solving together.[38] Meals and special foods are often an important element in celebrations such as birthdays and weddings, and they are a significant part of holiday traditions. These rituals may provide a sense of comfort, promote feelings of belonging, and offer respite from daily stressors. Mealtime participation can provide a predictable and positive context for parents to connect with children emotionally and to communicate family values and expectations, directly leading to greater well-being in children. Compared with family mealtime, other shared parent–child activities may not have the same potential for regularity, ritual, or focused time together.

However, the children with PFD face challenges in fully engaging and participating family meals. They may not be able to eat orally at all or may eat only small amounts of food due to lack of hunger, lack of feeding experience, or the clinician's concern about adverse consequences of oral feeding. Caregivers of children with SBS and other medical conditions can face an additional challenge in helping their children participate in regular family meals because the child's primary means of nutrition is often via PN and/or feeding tube. The time required for tube feedings and line care can interfere with caretaker time for organizing and planning the child's participation in mealtime.[39] When the child's medical needs negatively affect mealtimes, families lose a valuable and recurring opportunity for social contact and miss out on a sense of connectedness. Clinicians can help parents find ways to include their child with PFD in mealtime routines.

Practical application. Parents can include the older tube-fed child in family meals and mealtime routines in the following ways.

1. Have the child sit at the table during family meals. This gives the child who receives nutrition via PN or tube feeding the opportunity to become comfortable with the smells, tastes, textures, and routines of mealtime.
2. Provide the child with their own utensils and plate of food to taste, touch, and explore.
3. Encourage the child to help prepare food for mealtime. This has been shown to decrease food fussiness.[40]
4. Ask the child to set the table or contribute to other tasks that prepare for family mealtime.

Parent Education/Support

Strategy: parent responsive feeding
For both infants and children, the significance of the parent or caregiver's role in the feeding process cannot be overlooked when using strategies to promote oral feeding skills. Clinicians can educate parents about the importance of responsive feeding (RF), which involves identifying and appropriately responding to the child's satiety and hunger cues.

According to Berti and Agostoni, "RF consists of a mutual relationship between an infant or child and his/her caregiver: the caregiver creates routine, structure and emotional context that promote interaction; the child communicates feelings of hunger and satiety through motor actions, facial expressions, or vocalization; the caregiver immediately responds by providing appropriate and nutritious food in an emotionally and developmentally supportive manner, while maintaining an appropriate feeding environment; the child experiences predictable responses."[41]

The RF approach requires a caregiver to be sensitive and attentive to a child's hunger cues, such as rooting, sucking, or fussiness, then offering nutrition promptly and predictably. It is important to note that the way in which a parent offers food may impact the child's acceptance of it. The RF strategy allows a child to self-regulate their intake so they are being fed when genuinely hungry, which promotes their sense of autonomy and a positive experience with food. In addition, the mutual participation in RF cultivates trust and strengthens the bond between the caregiver and child, allowing for a more relaxed and positive attitude toward food.

In a systematic review, Howe and Wang concluded that "parent-directed and educational interventions for children with feeding problems are moderately to strongly effective in improving children's physical growth and development, increasing the feeding competence of children and their primary caretakers and improving parent-child interaction."[42] Morag and colleagues found that parents who used RF with infants who had nasogastric tubes reached full oral feeding within a shorter period of time, showed good weight gain, and were discharged home significantly earlier.[43]

Practical application. Clinicians can educate caregivers in the following basic RF strategies.

1. *Create a calm feeding environment:* Establish a quiet, distraction-free space for feeding that minimizes disruptions. This helps the child focus on their meal and allows parents to better tune into the child's signals.
2. *Learn hunger and fullness cues:* Familiarize themselves with the hunger and fullness cues specific to their child's age. Understanding these cues, such as sucking, rooting, or turning away from the spoon, allows parents to respond appropriately to their child's needs.
3. *Offer a variety of healthy foods:* Introduce a diverse range of nutritious foods to expose children to different tastes and textures. Be patient if a child initially rejects certain foods, as it may take multiple exposures (eg, 10–20) before they accept new flavors.

Learning to Eat by Mouth: A Case Study of a Young Girl with Short Bowel Syndrome

Introduction
This case study presents the journey of Emily, a young girl with SBS, who successfully transitioned from PN to oral feeding through a combination of medical intervention, some of the feeding strategies discussed in this article, and family support.

Medical history
Emily was born prematurely at 26 weeks gestation to young parents with a high school education and weighed only 1.2 kg at birth. Shortly after birth, she developed severe NEC, which necessitated multiple surgeries and major resections of her small bowel and colon. She was left with 65 cm of small bowel and one-half of her colon. A gastrostomy tube was not placed.

Background
Emily had an initial feeding and swallowing assessment by an occupational therapist while she was in the NICU. The occupational therapy (OT) found that she had good oral motor skills and her swallowing seemed safe. When the intestinal rehabilitation team felt she was ready for enteral feeds, Emily started receiving small volumes of expressed breast milk via bottle. The flow rate and positioning during feeding were adjusted to ensure the safety of oral feeds. The volume was gradually increased according to her stool output, limiting feeds to a volume that led to stool output of no more than 30 to 40 mL/kg/d. Emily's parents were informed about the complexity of

her condition and the need for long-term PN to ensure her growth and development before hospital discharge. They were educated in how to provide home PN care by the nursing staff and spent 24 hours in hospital providing their daughter's care under nursing supervision. Emily was discharged home on PN and small-volume oral feedings of breast milk.

After discharge, Emily continued to take the small volumes by mouth. She was not vomiting. Her intestine needed time to adapt, which meant that her tolerance for oral feeding was initially limited and increases in the volume of feedings given was slow. Following initial hospital discharge, the family faced numerous challenges, including frequent hospitalizations for complications related to PN, and they felt overwhelmed by the daunting challenge of teaching Emily to eat by mouth.

At 7 months of age, Emily's parents, with guidance from the multidisciplinary team, started introducing small tastes and amounts of pureed food. She was also transitioned from breast milk to a 20 cal/oz elemental infant formula. Her parents closely monitored her reactions and adjustments to her oral feeding plan were made as needed.

As a wider variety of tastes and textures were attempted, Emily demonstrated feeding aversion manifested by limited variety in her diet, gagging when presented with new foods, and decreased ability to chew textured foods. The multidisciplinary team recommended feeding therapy. Emily was referred to a pediatric occupational therapist who specialized in working with children with feeding difficulties who have complex medical conditions. The therapist conducted a comprehensive assessment of Emily's feeding abilities and challenges, considering factors such as oral motor skills, sensory aversions, and psychological barriers. The assessment revealed delayed oral motor skills, intraoral hypersensitivity, and anxiety when presented with novel foods.

Emily began weekly feeding therapy sessions that focused on oral motor skill development, introductions to food textures and tastes, and establishing a positive mealtime environment using RF practices. During therapy sessions, her parents were trained how to use games and play to help develop oral motor skills. They were provided with information on how to change the way foods are presented and encouraged to offer foods many times in a variety of ways. To help her parents establish positive mealtime experiences, they were provided information on how to use the Satter Division of Responsibility in Feeding. This encourages parents to determine what is served, when the meal or snack happens, and where the meals take place, while giving the child the choice of how much is eaten and whether it will be eaten at all.[44] The sessions were adjusted according to Emily's progress and tolerance of enteral feedings.

Challenges

- *Feeding aversion:* Emily initially exhibited feeding aversions, likely stemming from her past traumatic experiences related to intensive care, NEC, and surgical interventions.
- *Gastrointestinal adaptation:* Emily's remaining intestine needed time to adapt to feedings, which meant that her tolerance for oral feeding was initially limited.
- *Parental stress:* Emily's parents faced emotional stress and uncertainty throughout the process, as they had to manage her complex medical needs while teaching her to eat by mouth.

Results

- *Gradual progress:* Over several months, Emily made gradual progress in accepting oral feeds. Initially, she would only tolerate small spoonfuls of pureed food, but with time and consistent efforts, she began to consume larger amounts.

As her oral motor skills improved, she was able to chew and swallow age-appropriate foods.

- *Gastrointestinal adaptation:* Emily's remaining small intestine adapted well to the advancement of oral feeds. She experienced fewer complications related to SBS, gradually reducing the need for PN and achieving enteral autonomy by 24 months of age.
- *Improved quality of life:* As Emily became more proficient in eating by mouth, became less dependent on PN and her parents became more proficient in her care, the frequency of her hospitalizations decreased, and her parents reported improvements in her overall well-being and quality of life, as well as theirs.

Discussion

Emily's case highlights the importance of a multidisciplinary approach to treating children with SBS and other complex medical conditions. The combination of medical management, feeding therapy, and parental support was essential in helping Emily transition from reliance on PN to successful oral feeding. It also underscores the resilience and determination of young patients and their families in the face of complex medical conditions.

Conclusion

The journey of Emily, a young girl with SBS, showcases the potential for children with complex medical conditions to learn to eat by mouth using the strategies discussed in this article, along with appropriate medical guidance, comprehensive feeding and swallowing assessments, and dedicated parental involvement.

SUMMARY

Children with a history of ongoing intestinal failure are commonly at risk for feeding problems. For such children, oral feeding may have been impossible early in life, leading to challenges in achieving enteral autonomy through oral feeding. Additional factors challenging oral feeding are prior experiences with feeding or intubation that cause feeding aversion, as well as of the need for parental education and support in how to help the child with a feeding disorder at home. In these cases, children benefit from a multidisciplinary approach that considers the medical, anatomic, psychological, and social factors at play in pediatric feeding disorders. Members of such a care team can use several practical strategies to promote oral feeding in infants and children, including introducing oral feeding early/during the "critical window," using oral stimulation techniques when oral feeding is not possible, introducing complementary feeding at the appropriate age and timing, facilitating ways for a child to participate in mealtime even if they are not able to orally feed, and educating parents in RF techniques so they can build a trusting feeding relationship with their child and help them cultivate a positive attitude toward food and feeding.

CLINICS CARE POINTS

- After intestinal failure, watch for "red flags" (eg, choking or gagging, refusing to eat certain textures, negative behavior at mealtimes) that signal a child may need more support/additional strategies to successfully develop oral feeding skills.
- In infants, introducing oral feeding in the critical window of the first year of life is a crucial factor for later success. If oral feeding is not possible, oral stimulation and nonnutritive sucking are beneficial.

- Introducing complementary feeds as close as possible to developmentally appropriate times, using a variety of textures and flavors, and intentionally including children in family mealtime, despite feeding challenges, are essential practices for children with pediatric feeding disorder.
- When assessing a child with a feeding problem, keep in mind that the feeding relationship between child and caregiver may be a contributing factor.
- Parent education and support are crucial for promoting the success of oral feeding in children, and educating parents in responsive feeding techniques in particular yields benefits in a child's feeding and general attitude toward food.

DISCLOSURE

The authors have nothing to disclose.

REFERENCES

1. Carruth BR, Ziegler PJ, Gordon A, et al. Prevalence of picky eaters among infants and toddlers and their caregivers' decisions about offering a new food. J Am Diet Assoc 2004;104:57–64.
2. Manikam R, Perman JA. Pediatric feeding disorders. J Clin Gastroenterol 2000; 30:34–46.
3. Taylor CM, Wernimont SM, Northstone K, et al. Picky/fussy eating in children: Review of definitions, assessment, prevalence and dietary intakes. Appetite 2015; 95:349–59.
4. Park J, Thoyre SM, Pados BF, et al. Symptoms of feeding problems in preterm-born children at 6 months to 7 years old. J Pediatr Gastroenterol Nutr 2019; 68(3):416–21.
5. Gigola F, Carletti V, Coletta R, et al. Treatment of food aversion and eating problems in children with short bowel syndrome: a systematic review. Children 2022; 9(10):1582.
6. Christian VJ, Van Hoorn M, Walia CLS, et al. Pediatric feeding disorder in children with short bowel syndrome. J Pediatr Gastroenterol Nutr 2021;72:442–5.
7. Goday PS, Huh SY, Silverman A, et al. Pediatric feeding disorder: Consensus definition and conceptual framework. J Pediatr Gastroenterol Nutr 2019;68: 124–9.
8. Yang CF, Duro D, Zurakowski D, et al. High prevalence of multiple micronutrient deficiencies in children with intestinal failure: a longitudinal study. J Pediatr 2011; 159:39–44.
9. Pironi L, Arends J, Baxter J, et al. ESPEN endorsed recommendations. Definition and classification of intestinal failure in adults. Clin Nutr 2015;34:171–80.
10. Modi BP, Galloway DP, Gura K, et al. ASPEN definitions in pediatric intestinal failure. J Parenter Enteral 2022;46(1):42–59.
11. Merritt RJ, Cohran V, Raphael BP, et al. Intestinal rehabilitation programs in the management of pediatric intestinal failure and short bowel syndrome. J Pediatr Gastroenterol Nutr 2017;65:588–96.
12. Belza C, Patterson C, Ghent E, et al. "Line care governs our entire world": Understanding the experience of caregivers of children with intestinal failure receiving long-term parenteral nutrition. JPEN - J Parenter Enter Nutr 2022;46:1602–13.
13. Belza C, Avitzur Y, Ungar WJ, et al. Stress, anxiety, depression, and health-related quality of life in caregivers of children with intestinal failure receiving

parenteral nutrition: A cross-sectional survey study. JPEN - J Parenter Enter Nutr 2023;47:342–53.

14. Bondi BC, Gold A, Belza C, et al. Predictors of social-emotional development and adaptive functioning in school-age children with intestinal failure. J Clin Psychol Med Settings 2023;30:589–605.

15. Gold A, Danguecan A, Belza C, et al. Neurocognitive functioning in early school-age children with intestinal failure. J Pediatr Gastroenterol Nutr 2020;70:225–31.

16. Bell M, Cole CR, Hansen NI, et al. Neurodevelopmental and growth outcomes of extremely preterm infants with short bowel syndrome. J Pediatr 2021;230: 76–83.e5.

17. Gateau K, Song A, Vanderbilt DL, et al. Maternal post-traumatic stress and depression symptoms and outcomes after NICU discharge in a low-income sample: a cross-sectional study. BMC Pregnancy Childbirth 2021;21:48.

18. Boctor DL, Jutteau WH, Fenton TR, et al. The prevalence of feeding difficulties and potential risk factors in pediatric intestinal failure: Time to consider promoting oral feeds. Clin Nutr 2021;40:5399–406.

19. Katzman DK, Norris ML, Zucker N. Avoidant restrictive food intake disorder. Psychiatr Clin North Am 2019;42:45–57.

20. Zickgraf HF, Lane-Loney S, Essayli JH, et al. Further support for diagnostically meaningful ARFID symptom presentations in an adolescent medicine partial hospitalization program. Int J Eat Disord 2019;52:402–9.

21. Białek-Dratwa A, Szymańska D, Grajek M, et al. ARFID—Strategies for dietary management in children. Nutrients 2022;14(9):1739.

22. Homan GJ. Failure to thrive: a practical guide. Am Fam Physician 2016;94(4): 295–9.

23. Kessler DB, Dawson PE. Failure to thrive and pediatric undernutrition: a transdisciplinary approach. Baltimore, MD: Brookes; 1999.

24. Tang MN, Adolphe S, Rogers SR, et al. Failure to thrive or growth faltering: Medical, developmental/behavioral, nutritional, and social dimensions. Pediatr Rev 2021;42(11):590–603.

25. Becker P, Carney LN, Corkins MR, et al. Consensus statement of the Academy of Nutrition and Dietetics/American Society for Parenteral and Enteral Nutrition: indicators recommended for the identification and documentation of pediatric malnutrition (undernutrition). Nutr Clin Pract 2015;30:147–61.

26. Mehta NM, Corkins MR, Lyman B, et al. Defining pediatric malnutrition: a paradigm shift toward etiology-related definitions. JPEN - J Parenter Enter Nutr 2013;37:460–81.

27. Kerzner B, Milano K, MacLean WC Jr, et al. A practical approach to classifying and managing feeding difficulties. Pediatrics 2015;135(2):344–53.

28. Goulet O, Olieman J, Ksiazyk J, et al. Neonatal short bowel syndrome as a model of intestinal failure: physiological background for enteral feeding. Clin Nutr 2013; 32(2):162–71.

29. Norsa L, Goulet O, Alberti D, et al. Nutrition and intestinal rehabilitation of children with short bowel syndrome: a position paper of the ESPGHAN Committee on Nutrition. Part 1: from intestinal resection to home discharge. J Pediatr Gastroenterol Nutr 2023;77(2):281–97.

30. Hopkins J, Cermak SA, Merritt RJ. Oral feeding difficulties in children with short bowel syndrome: a narrative review. Nutr Clin Pract 2018;33(1):99–106.

31. Calk P. Best practices for oral motor stimulation to improve oral feeding in preterm infants: a systematic review. Ann Physiother Occup Ther 2019;2(5).

32. Li L, Liu L, Chen F, et al. Clinical effects of oral motor intervention combined with non-nutritive sucking on oral feeding in preterm infants with dysphagia. J Pediatr 2022;98(6):635–40.
33. Fucile S, Gisele E, McFarland D, et al. Oral and non-oral sensorimotor interventions enhance oral feeding performance in preterm infants. Dev Med Child Neurol 2011;53(9):829–35.
34. Mennella JA, Trabulsi JC. Complementary foods and flavor experiences: setting the foundation. Ann Nutr Metab 2012;60(Suppl 2):40–50.
35. Coulthard H, Harris G, Emmett P. Delayed introduction of lumpy foods to children during the complementary feeding period affects child's food acceptance and feeding at 7 years of age. Matern Child Nutr 2009;5(1):75–85.
36. Verlato G, Hill S, Jonkers-Schuitema C, et al. Results of an international survey on feeding management in infants with short bowel syndrome-associated intestinal failure. J Pediatr Gastroenterol Nutr 2020;73(5):647–53.
37. Case-Smith J. Systematic reviews of the effectiveness of interventions used in occupational therapy early childhood services. Am J Occup Ther 2013;67(4): 379–82.
38. Fiese B, Foley K, Spagnola M. Routine and ritual elements in family mealtimes: contexts for child well-being and family identity. N Dir Child Adolesc Dev 2006; 111:67–89.
39. Winston K. Feeding a child with mealtime challenges: a mother's work. Work 2015;50(3):443–50.
40. Chilman L, Kennedy-Behr A, Frakking T, et al. Picky eating in children: A scoping review to examine its intrinsic and extrinsic features and how they relate to identification. Int J Environ Res Publ Health 2021;17(18):9067.
41. Berti C, Agostoni C. Establishing healthy eating patterns in infancy. In: Saavedra JM, editor. Dattilo AM. Early nutrition and long-term health. 2nd edition. Sawston, UK: Woodhead; 2022. p. 493–535.
42. Howe T, Wang T. Systematic review of interventions used in or relevant to occupational therapy for children with feeding difficulties ages birth–5 years. Am J Occup Ther 2013;67(4):405–12.
43. Morag I, Hendel Y, Karol D, et al. Transition from nasogastric tube to oral feeding: the role of parental guided responsive feeding. Front pediatr 2019;7(190). https://doi.org/10.3389/fped.2019.00190.
44. Satter E. Child of mine: feeding with love and good sense. Michigan: Bull Publishing; 1986. https://openlibrary.org/books/OL17988809M/Child_of_mine.

Moving?

Make sure your subscription moves with you!

To notify us of your new address, find your **Clinics Account Number** (located on your mailing label above your name), and contact customer service at:

Email: journalscustomerservice-usa@elsevier.com

800-654-2452 (subscribers in the U.S. & Canada)
314-447-8871 (subscribers outside of the U.S. & Canada)

Fax number: 314-447-8029

**Elsevier Health Sciences Division
Subscription Customer Service
3251 Riverport Lane
Maryland Heights, MO 63043**

*To ensure uninterrupted delivery of your subscription, please notify us at least 4 weeks in advance of move.

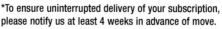